After obtaining a degree in zoology and teaching in schools and colleges, Oliver Cowmeadow encountered Eastern philosophy and medicine in 1980. Immediatcly taken by the Oriental view of life and health, he studied the Eastern philosophy and its application in Shiatsu and macrobiotics intensively in London, Boston and Europe.

Oliver has been practising Shiatsu and giving dietary consultations in the South West of England since 1983. He currently practises in Devon and is the principal of the Devon School of Shiatsu, running introductory and professional training courses in Shiatsu. This is his fifth book on the Eastern approach to healthcare.

Other books in *A Practical Introduction* series:

Tai Chi by Paul Crompton
Reflexology and Colour Therapy by Pauline Wills
Yoga by Dr Svami Purna

Shiatsu

A PRACTICAL INTRODUCTION

Oliver Cowmeadow

ELEMENT

Shaftesbury, Dorset ● Boston, Massachusetts
Melbourne, Victoria

First published as *The Art of Shiatsu* in the UK in 1992 by
Element Books Limited

This edition first published in the UK in 1998 by Element Books Limited
Shaftesbury, Dorset SP7 8BP

Published in the USA in 1998 by Element, Inc
160 North Washington Street, Boston, MA 02114

Published in Australia in 1998 by Element Books
and distributed by Penguin Australia Limited
487 Maroondah Highway, Ringwood, Victoria 3134

Cover design by Slatter-Anderson
Illustrations by David Woodroffe
Diagrams by Phil Payter Graphics
Designed by Linda Reed and Associates
Printed and bound in Great Britain by
Butler & Tanner Ltd, Frome and London

British Library Cataloguing in Publication data available

Library of Congress Cataloging in Publication data available

ISBN 1 86204 162 8

Contents

Preface   1

How to Use this Book   2

A Note on Nomenclature   2

Author's Note   3

Part 1 **Shiatsu and Energy**   5
  1. What is Shiatsu?   6
  2. Our Energetic Constitution   12
  3. Exercises to Perceive Ki   30

Part 2 **Learning to Give Shiatsu**   37
  4. Practical Details   38
  5. Preliminary Exercises   45
  6. A Basic Shiatsu Sequence   58

Part 3 **Developing Your Shiatsu Further**   85
  7. Adapting Your Shiatsu for Different People 86
  8. The Next Step – Kyo and Jitsu   88
  9. The Energetics of Food   93
  10. Oriental Diagnosis and Body Reading 108
  11. Incorporating Tsubos into your Shiatsu 126
  12. Meridian Exercises for Yourself 139

Postscript   147

Glossary   148

Further Reading   150

Useful Addresses   151

Index   152

Preface

This book has a dual purpose. Firstly it intends to introduce a different way of seeing the world and ourselves, based on the Energetic nature of life. While many traditional cultures have recognized the Energetic basis of life and health, modern Western culture has almost exclusively focused on the material aspect. Gaining a perception and knowledge of the human Energetic make-up opens up new possibilities for understanding our health and how to alleviate health problems.

Secondly, this book gives a comprehensive guide for the beginner to learn the healing art of Shiatsu, a system of healing that primarily works on an Energetic level. It is a practical method of learning to perceive the Energetic nature of the human body and being, and to use Energy to promote health and alleviate sickness.

Although the roots of Shiatsu are very old, it has developed a great deal this century, gaining from the contributions of a number of different sources of wisdom. While based on traditional Chinese medicine, it has been enriched and extended by modern Shiatsu teachers like Toru Namikoshi and Shizuto Masunaga in Japan and Wataru Ohashi in the West, by the modern Western understanding of anatomy and physiology, and by macrobiotic teachings which combine a traditional Eastern understanding of life and health with the modern Western scientific understanding.

While everyone giving Shiatsu is using the same basic ideas and technique, the variety of sources of knowledge and techniques used in Shiatsu has created a number of different styles. This book represents my particular style, drawn from traditional Shiatsu teachings, macrobiotics and other sources on the nature of our subtle Energetic being. It will give a sound foundation in understanding and giving Shiatsu, and can be used as a basis for further study in any style you may later encounter.

How to Use this Book

The format of this book is based on the many introductory Shiatsu classes that I have taught in Devon and Cornwall. It is designed as a step-by-step guide, to be read and used in sequence chapter by chapter. Part 1 gives an introduction to the approach of Shiatsu and our Energetic make-up. This section can be quite quickly read through and the exercises to perceive Energy practised.

The chapters of Part 2 are practical in nature and give instruction on learning to give Shiatsu. After working through these chapters you may want to read no further, and keep using this section over a few weeks to perfect your ability to give an effective full-body Shiatsu treatment.

Part 3 contains a lot of extra information to experiment with for months to come. While you might be drawn to reading through them earlier on, each one primarily gives information to be practically applied in your giving of Shiatsu and in your daily life. As such, they will take time to digest and assimilate. *Bon appetit*!

A Note on Nomenclature

In this book some words begin with a capital letter, to show that they are being used to represent an Oriental concept. For example, 'Energy' refers to the Oriental idea of subtle energy which is different from the usual Western idea of 'energy', and 'Kidneys' refers to an Oriental concept which is different from the Western scientific understanding of the kidneys as physical organs. These Oriental concepts will be explained in the text of the book, but you can also refer to the Glossary on page 148 for brief definitions.

Author's Note

This book is not meant to be used as a substitute for professional medical help. Please consult a doctor or other qualified health practitioner if you are in any doubt about the cause and treatment of any health problem.

Dedication

I would like to thank all the teachers who have contributed so much to my learning about life, especially Michio and Aveline Kushi, Saul Goodman and Denny Waxman, together with all my friends and colleagues with whom I share this adventure.

PART 1

Shiatsu and Energy?

CHAPTER 1

What is Shiatsu?

The word 'Shiatsu' is Japanese and literally means 'finger pressure', as this is the main technique used in giving Shiatsu. Pressure is also applied to the body with the palms of the hands, and sometimes with the elbows, knees and feet to give stronger pressure. Stretching exercises are also applied to increase flexibility in a similar way to yoga or other loosening-up exercises.

Shiatsu could be said to be a combination of acupuncture and massage. Like the ancient Chinese art of acupuncture, Shiatsu works on the flow of Chi, Ki or 'Life Energy' that circulates through the body in specific channels or Meridians. By promoting the steady and unimpeded flow of Ki and rebalancing the flow where it has become either excessive or deficient, health is increased and many health problems alleviated. However, rather than inserting needles into the body, Shiatsu uses touch with the hands or other parts of the body. As with massage, this touch by another human can have great healing effects in itself. We have all put a hand over a knock or a painful part of the body to relieve pain, or have experienced how much the holding of a hand or an arm around the shoulder can relieve suffering. Shiatsu is like a specialized system of touching that will have the greatest healing effects.

A Brief History of Shiatsu

The foundation of Shiatsu lies in ancient Chinese medicine. The earliest recorded writing on Chinese medicine, *The Yellow Emperor's Classic of Internal Medicine*, written over 2000 years ago, contains a wealth of information on the causes of many illnesses and how they may be remedied using changes in diet and life style and with acupuncture and massage. This ancient Oriental medicine has been greatly enlarged and developed over the last 2000 years. The Chinese form of massage found its way to Japan, where it was called Anma. Anma was often practised by blind people, and was widely used to treat common ailments.

During this century in Japan, new influences on Anma from both the traditions of the East and modern Western science shaped it into what is now called Shiatsu. About twenty years ago, Shiatsu began spreading to the West where it has caught on with amazing rapidity. In Britain, early students of Shiatsu have been instrumental in setting up a number of schools offering professional courses in Shiatsu, so that the number of qualified Shiatsu therapists is rapidly increasing. In the last few years a lot of media coverage has brought the benefits of Shiatsu to the public's attention, and it is gaining wide acceptance as a powerful and effective therapy.

Eastern and Western Medicine

In many ways the philosophical approaches to life and health are opposite in the East and West. This does not necessarily mean that they are in conflict with each other or cannot be used side by side, but rather that they take a very different view of health and sickness. In fact, these two opposite approaches complement each other very well, as do all opposites.

One particular opposite viewpoint of these two great efforts to understand health and cure sickness is that modern Western medicine studies the physical or material functioning of the body such as its mechanical working and chemical nature, whereas traditional Eastern medicine primarily sought to understand the Energetic basis of life, health and disease. This Energy is called Chi in Chinese, Ki in Japanese, and Prana in India, and has been called 'Life Energy', 'Orgone Energy' or 'Subtle Energy' in the West. It is not the same as the Western scientific idea of energy, which is based on the energetic content of physical matter, such as the amount of heat produced by the burning of food measured in calories or joules. Rather, it is believed that a more subtle form of Energy pervades the whole universe, and that from this universal Energy, matter is formed. Living organisms are seen as particularly active centres of subtle Energy, their very life depending on constant nourishment not only by the physical nutrients but also by this Energy.

So far no scientific instruments have been able directly to detect or measure subtle Energy, although some instruments can detect it indirectly by measuring skin resistance to find acupuncture points over the body. This Energy can be felt quite easily by other living organisms, and anyone can learn to perceive it for themselves. (The exercises in Chapter 3 will enable you to do so.)

Shiatsu, like acupuncture, affects a particular system of Energy in the body; that of the Meridians. *Meridian* is a French word (acupuncture was first introduced from the East to France) meaning 'channel', and describes the channels of Energy which flow over the surface of the body and into the interior of the body to the Organs. The surface part of the Meridians offers an easy way to affect the flow of Energy through all of the body by simple touch, or through the insertion of needles as in acupuncture, or through the application of heat as in moxibustion. These efforts to affect Energy flow in the Meridians are often centred on particular points along the Meridians which have been found to be especially effective. These are known as acupuncture or acupressure points, or as Tsubos in Japanese.

The Role of Shiatsu Today

Shiatsu has two main applications or roles in society today. Firstly as a therapy offered by qualified practitioners who have studied the subject in depth, and secondly by anyone who has studied Shiatsu a little from books or in short courses in order to relax family members and friends and deal with minor health problems. Let's look at Shiatsu as a therapy first.

The rapid rise in popularity of Shiatsu would suggest that there is a great need for it at this time. One of the main reasons for this is that it is effective in remedying many problems which Western medicine can do little for. For example, many people suffer from problems in which no physical changes can be found in the blood, body chemistry or body structure. Orthodox medicine can therefore offer little or nothing to remedy the problem, except perhaps a palliative to remove the pain or other symptom. Some examples are cases of back pain, headaches, migraines, other aches, pains or chronic tension in the body, insomnia, irregularities in menstrual cycles or painful periods, low libido or vitality, and prevalent negative moods like depression, anxiety or worry.

Shiatsu, with its basis of Oriental medicine, has the means to understand how certain definite imbalances in Energy create these kinds of problems, and can therefore often alleviate them. On many occasions I have seen clients who have been told that physically there is nothing wrong with them but who nevertheless have various 'minor' ailments which interfere with their living a normal happy life. Sometimes the inner feelings of the client are vague, such as feeling weak in the legs, especially when having to stand and talk in front of people, or having an 'empty head' with an inability to think clearly or remember simple things, and the lack of acknowledgement that something is definitely wrong has left them thinking they may be a little mad.

In these cases clients are enormously relieved when assured that the symptoms are definitely real and can be perfectly explained by Oriental theory. A single treatment or a series of weekly treatments is very often effective in eradicating this type of problem.

Besides giving the actual treatment, most shiatsu practitioners also give advice on how clients may themselves do things to help improve their health and alleviate their problems. This may take the form of changes in diet, specific exercises to practise, more regular exercise, or changes in a person's life style.

Often people go to a Shiatsu therapist to remedy a specific problem, but over a number of treatments they may also experience other benefits, such as sleeping more deeply, feeling calmer, more centred and less uptight, feeling lighter and brighter, or the disappearance of old aches and pains. In fact some people will visit a Shiatsu therapist regularly just for these more general health benefits. This highlights the fact that as well as being an effective remedy for many specific health problems, Shiatsu also promotes overall health of the body, mind and spirit. In this way it acts preventively, reducing the chances of a person becoming ill in the future.

Then Shiatsu can also be learned at a basic level by anyone for their own benefit and for that of their family and friends. At this level, one would not gain the knowledge to help with many of the more serious problems that a qualified Shiatsu therapist may be able to deal with. Nevertheless, even after just a little study and practise the benefits to the receiver can be great. After attending an introductory class, many students have reported helping relieve friends' minor backaches, knee problems, aching shoulders, insomnia and other problems. And then there are the wider benefits of having tension and stress removed from the body, calming the nervous system, increasing energy and a greater sense of aliveness that comes from a better overall flow of Energy through the Meridians.

Can Anyone Learn to Give Shiatsu?

Yes! You don't have to have any special abilities to be able to learn Shiatsu, and anyone can learn to sense Energy in time. Obviously some people may learn a little more quickly, especially those who have had some experience in massage or other forms of bodywork or in healing, but virtually anyone can learn to give effective Shiatsu. One advantage of Shiatsu is that it does not require great muscular strength and is not physically taxing to give. So children, older people or lightly built people can give Shiatsu as effectively as more athletic types.

The Benefits of Learning Shiatsu

These are some of the benefits and joys that learning Shiatsu can bring.

1 In learning Shiatsu you learn more about your own health and how you can improve it, as well as how to remedy many common problems and help prevent future illness.

2 Shiatsu is such a simple way of healing, just using the hands, which we carry with us everywhere! So you can offer your healing help at almost any time and in any place. Practically everyone enjoys receiving Shiatsu and benefits from the deep relaxation and healing it brings.

3 In Shiatsu we heal with our caring touch. It is a way of communicating our love and compassion for others in a very direct way. Giving Shiatsu to our family and friends is a wonderful way of nourishing others and strengthening our relationships.

4 Giving Shiatsu is an uplifting experience. By the giving of our Energy, we receive more Energy. When Shiatsu is given in a calm, relaxed and compassionate way, the giver feels physically, mentally and spiritually uplifted and Energized. This contrasts with many activities which tire us by using up our Energy.

5 If you can, learn to give Shiatsu with a friend so that you can practise on each other. You will then receive Shiatsu regularly, which is a great help in your learning of Shiatsu, and also means that you will receive its healing benefits.

6 If you enjoy giving Shiatsu you may well consider practising it as a career. Since the introduction of Shiatsu to Britain about sixteen years ago, many schools have opened all over the country, training people to give Shiatsu professionally (a list of schools is given at the end of the book). If you discover a strong attraction to this healing art, you may wish to study Shiatsu to reach a professional level.

7 Shiatsu is a potent method of self-development. It has many similarities to other Eastern methods of personal development such as aikido, tai chi, chi kung, yoga and meditation. In learning Shiatsu one develops many inner qualities that are equally useful in the rest of one's life. These include becoming more centred, grounded and able to stay calm and relaxed while busy or under pressure, developing a greater sensitivity to other people and perception of their health, moods and thoughts, calming of the mind and enhanced intuition.

Usually I give Shiatsu treatments every week. Occasionally I am involved in other work and do not give any for a while. I so miss the unique experience of giving Shiatsu that I end up dying to get my hands on someone, and when I do, I feel so much better! You too may get bitten by the Shiatsu bug and end up an addict. It is my sincere wish that you do.

CHAPTER 2

Our Energetic Constitution

In giving Shiatsu, we are primarily working with our own and another person's Energy. Those of us brought up in modern Western culture are generally quite unaware of the Energetic nature of life. In contrast, most developed Eastern cultures in past millennia clearly perceived Energy as the basis of life. For example, in India it was called Prana, in China Chi and in Japan Ki. In the ancient languages of these countries their word for Energy crops up in all kinds of phrases and expressions; it was an integral part of their understanding of their lives and the universe. Yet most languages of Western societies do not even have a word for this Energy. In recent times various words have come into use, such as 'Life Energy', 'Orgone Energy', and 'Vital Energy'. In the rest of this book, Ki or simply Energy will be used.

Because Ki is so little recognized in our modern, materially orientated culture, you will probably have little or no experience of perceiving it. Don't lose heart! Everyone can learn to perceive Ki, and appreciate how it is an integral part of life. Learning the art of Shiatsu is an excellent way of learning to perceive Ki. With time and practice the world of Ki can become every bit as definite as the physical world. To help you appreciate the world of Ki, it may be helpful to describe briefly the Oriental understanding of the nature of the universe.

Figure 1 illustrates the relationship between the physical, Energetic and spiritual worlds. In the last couple of centuries Western culture has focused on the scientific investigation of the material world, and seeks to explain the nature of life and health in material terms. In contrast, Oriental cultures have looked more at the Energetic world, which is seen as being much larger and encompassing the world of matter.

Matter is seen as the most condensed form of Energy, with a continual interchange of Energy condensing to form matter and matter disintegrating to form Energy. This idea or observation has been demonstrated to some extent by modern physics, which has produced the disintegration of atoms into energy and the formation of atomic particles by energy.

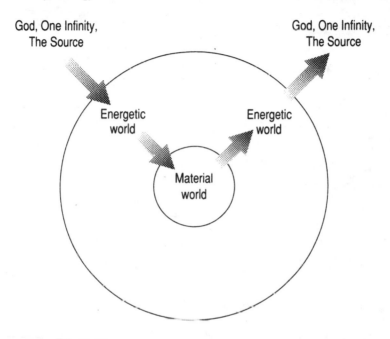

Fig. 1 The Relationship between Matter and Energy

The modern Western concept of energy is associated with matter, such as the number of calories that food will produce when fully burned up. Other forms of energy include various types of electromagnetic energy such as light, X-rays and radio waves. The Eastern concept of Energy is quite distinct from this more physical form of energy. It is of a more subtle nature that is easily perceived by living organisms such as human beings but is yet to be measured by a scientific instrument, although this may well happen in the future.

And where does Energy come from? The idea of God, One Infinity, The Source or a state of Absolute Oneness is universal and has been given different names in different cultures. This state is the source of

Energy, matter and life, and at the same time encompasses all Energy, matter and phenomena. The aim of religions and philosophies world-wide has been to raise human consciousness to appreciate God or the Absolute state. Raising our awareness to appreciate the world of Energy is a step in this direction.

In this traditional view, life is created by Energy. Organized patterns of Energy create an organized physical body, and our emotions, feelings, thoughts and other levels of consciousness are particular manifestations of Energy. When there is abundant Energy, there is aliveness. When Energy is weak or absent, there is lifelessness. So if we want to understand life, we need to understand Energy!

In the rest of this chapter we will briefly survey the major systems of Energy that make up our being, to give a comprehensive idea of our Energetic constitution. In many traditional cultures, people's aware-ness of Energy was much greater and they described several major systems of Energy in the human body. As we become more sensitive to Energy, we too can perceive these Energy systems and confirm their presence to ourselves. You may already be familiar with some of them. In particular, the Oriental systems of Organs, Meridians and Tsubos, which are most used in Shiatsu, will be introduced.

The Subtle Body System

Many teachings from around the world, including yoga teachings, vedantic scriptures, theosophical knowledge and Western researchers, describe a number of subtle Energetic bodies in addition to the physical body. These subtle Energetic bodies are seen as overlying the physical body and each other, and extending outside the physical boundary of the body to different distances to form the aura. Each is of a different frequency or 'fineness' of Energy and so maintains its integrity, just as a number of radio or television stations use different frequencies of radio waves and so do not interfere with each other.

The number of subtle bodies described varies a little, although there is general agreement on the denser Energetic bodies shown in Figure 2 on page 16.

The **etheric body** is the densest level of subtle Energy, and is close-ly associated with the functioning of the physical body. It extends a few inches beyond the skin and is probably what is detected by Kirlian photography. The Meridian and Organ systems described later probably exist mainly as part of the etheric body. The first two exercises in Chapter 3 will enable you to feel the etheric body around your hands and over another person. Many forms of healing using the hands work on the etheric level.

The **astral body** is of a higher frequency or finer level of subtle Energy than the etheric body, and extends several feet from the physical body. The astral body is the vehicle of our emotions and to the clairvoyant able to see it, it varies in shape and colour according to the emotions being experienced by a person.

Although the astral aura is more difficult to perceive directly, many daily experiences involve it. Interactions with other people are often primarily on an emotional level and bring about changes in the astral body. When strong emotions are being expressed, the Energy of those emotions gets picked up by the astral body and they may continue to be felt for some time. One may pick up on positive emotions like joy, courage or confidence, or negative emotions like doubt, depression or anger. A way to avoid picking up negative emotions is to be mentally conscious of the emotions being given out and to make the mental decision not to take on those emotions. One can then be open and sympathetic without the unfortunate consequence of taking on the other's negative emotions.

When two people meet they generally keep a certain safe distance from each other, maintaining their 'personal space', and to approach too closely feels uncomfortable. Basically, they stay just far enough away to avoid their astral bodies overlapping. Once two people feel safe with each other or have some emotional relationship, then the need to keep their astral bodies separated goes, and a hug or other close contact feels comfortable.

The **mental body** is composed of yet finer subtle Energy and extends further out from the physical body. It is the vehicle of the intellect or thinking mind and contains specific thoughtforms. To the clairvoyant able to perceive the mental aura, ideas and concepts that a person is conveying can be seen like pictures. It is also the medium of telepathy. When the mental body is developed, it allows an individual to think clearly and to focus mental energies with force and clarity.

The physical, etheric, astral and mental bodies together form a person's personality.

The **causal body** is also called the higher self or soul. It is composed of still finer subtle Energy and extends out far beyond the other bodies. It deals more with intuitive perceptions and understanding. Whereas the mental body is concerned more with analysing or dividing things up in order to understand them, the causal body is synthetic or wholistic, understanding the essence of things and their connection with the whole. In the reincarnation theory, it is considered that at death the physical, astral and mental bodies die while the casual body, or soul, continues on to new lives, where it takes on a new personality in order to develop itself further.

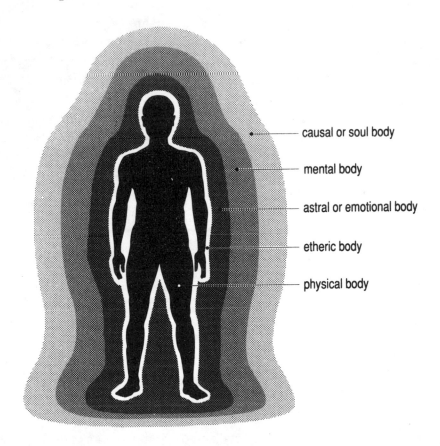

causal or soul body

mental body

astral or emotional body

etheric body

physical body

Fig. 2 The Physical and Energetic Bodies

In understanding health and healing a few points can be made on the interrelationships of our various subtle bodies. Firstly, these bodies contain our consciousness on different levels; consciousness of our body, emotions, thoughts and intuition. Our consciousness changes levels frequently as we shift our attention between these different levels, and so different subtle bodies are activated. During the process of maturing and personal development, a person's consciousness widens and the higher levels become more active. Whereas a young child is concerned mainly with its physical and emotional experience, in youth the mental faculties become more active, and in a mature adult intellectual and intuitive abilities become more developed.

Secondly, energy passes between the bodies, down to more materialized levels or up to finer levels. Therefore changes in the physical body will affect the etheric body and through that, the emotional, mental and causal bodies. That is to say, our physical health is the foundation of health at other levels. Likewise, our emotions or thoughts will have an effect on our physical body and affect our physical health, and events on a causal or soul level will affect all the other bodies or levels of our being.

Thirdly, from the foregoing it is clear that it is necessary to have a wide variety of healing methods to deal with all the different bodies. Modern scientifically orientated medicine primarily affects the physical body with its use of surgery, chemically based drugs, radiation therapy and so on. Many traditional healing methods primarily act on the etheric body, such as acupuncture and Shiatsu. Other traditional and modern approaches to healing are primarily directed at restoring to health or developing the emotional, mental and causal bodies.

Shiatsu techniques primarily work on the Meridians, which are a part of the etheric body, and through this level bring about changes on a physical, emotional and mental level. However, as an individual becomes more sensitive to Energy on other finer levels, they can also work directly on these.

The Spiritual Channel and the Chakras

The strongest flow of Energy in the body is in the spiritual channel or Sushumna, running from the top of the head to the base of the torso.

This channel is charged by Energy coming from above and below. When we think of ourselves just as a physical body, it seems that we are quite separate from anything outside our physical boundary, the skin. When we see ourselves as Energy, this separation disappears. We only exist because of the constant flow of Energy into us from other people, from the earth and other living organisms, from the sun, planets, stars and outer space.

When our body is erect, the flow of these two forces is greatest, increasing the activity of the physical body, the mind and spiritual awareness. Hence if you are reading a demanding book, playing a musical instrument or doing anything else that demands a great input of Energy, it is much easier if you sit up with a straight back rather than slumping

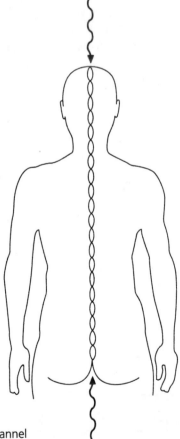

Fig. 3 The Spiritual Channel

or lying down. On the other hand if you want to relax it is better to lie down. A straight, upright posture has long been recognized as desirable for meditation. It also aids concentration, hence schoolteachers' sometimes frequent admonitions to 'sit up straight' and 'don't slouch'!

On the spiritual channel there are seven main centres of Energy, often called Chakras. **Chakra** is a Sanskrit word meaning 'wheel', as this is how they can appear to a clairvoyant. The Chakras are a part of the subtle Energy bodies. Each Chakra has an etheric component, nourishing the surrounding Organs and their functions, and also a specific endocrine gland producing hormones in the physical body. Each Chakra also has an astral or emotional component, a mental and a causal component, and so forms a centre of consciousness. The main functions of the seven Chakras are summarized in the table below.

Chakra	Gland	Physical organs and parts governed	Emotional, mental and spiritual functions
Crown	Pineal	Upper brain and right eye	Spiritual awareness, spiritual will-to-be
Ajna or Brow	Pituitary	Lower brain, left eye, ears, nose and nervous system	Higher mind, intuitive perception and understanding
Throat	Thyroid	Lungs, mouth, throat, vocal cords, shoulders, arms, hands and lymphatic system	Self-expression, communication, creativity
Heart	Thymus	Heart, circulatory system, Vagus nerve and breasts	Love, compassion, service to humanity, awareness of self
Solar Plexus	Pancreas	Stomach and digestive system, spleen, liver and gall bladder	Personal power, desire, source of emotions
Sacral	Gonads	Reproductive system, lower back, legs and feet	Physical and mental vitality, grounded-ness, sexual energy, relationships and self-esteem
Base	Adrenals	The spine and skeleton, kidneys, bladder and autonomic nervous system	Physical will-to-be and procreation

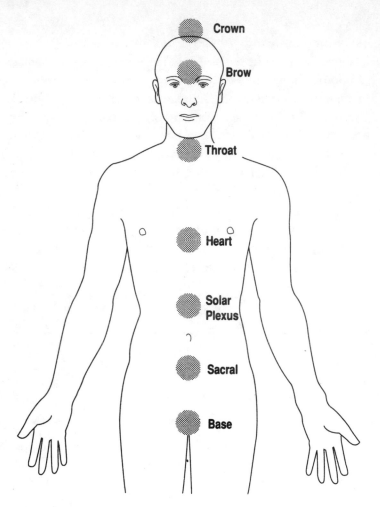

Fig. 4 The Seven Main Chakras

With the subtle bodies we saw that, with the development of consciousness over a lifetime, activity tends to shift to finer bodies, from the physical and etheric to the astral, mental and causal. A similar progression occurs in Chakra activity. While all the Chakras are active in supporting the physical functioning of the body, in emotional, mental and spiritual activity there is a development from the lower Chakras to the upper Chakras. The lowest three Chakras are concerned with our personal survival and our physical and emotional relations with other people and the outside world. The diaphragm can be thought of as a borderline between these 'lower' functions and our 'higher' human functions or qualities. The fourth and fifth Chakras, the heart and throat, become more active as individuals develop their ability to love and become creative in communicating ideas and concepts. With an increased intuitive understanding of the nature of life and the universe, the sixth brow Chakra becomes more active. The seventh crown Chakra only becomes fully active when people have developed their awareness, on a spiritual level, of the unity of all life. Thus every change in consciousness is reflected in a change in the activity of the Chakras.

As we saw with the subtle bodies, there is also a movement of Energy between the different subtle bodies within each Chakra. Therefore if there is a change at one level, this will tend to create changes in all the other bodies of the same Chakra. For example, if there is a physical problem, say in the throat, a person often, but not invariably, may also be suffering from a difficulty in expressing his or her inner feelings and thoughts.

The Oriental Concept of Organs

In Oriental medicine the Organs have a wider meaning based on their Energetic functions. For example, the Oriental idea of the Kidneys includes not only the physical kidneys and their function of controlling water metabolism, but also the Energetic functions of nourishing the bones, spine and brain, the ears and the hair, and creating willpower and memory. Therefore problems in any of these areas can be due to an imbalance in Kidney Energy.

Twelve main Organs are described in Chinese medicine. Six are concerned with the storage of Energy and are called Zang. The other six, called Fu, are concerned with *transforming* food and drink into Energy to be stored in the Zang, and with the excretion of waste products. The Zang are all 'solid' Organs such as the Liver, whereas the Fu are all 'hollow' Organs such as the Stomach.

Each of the Zang is paired with a Fu because of a similarity in function. The six pairs are shown in the table on page 22 together with their main functions. Note that the physical organ of the pancreas is generally considered to be included in the Spleen Organ. The Heart Governor and Triple Heater Organs do not have a direct physical counterpart as with the other Organs. The Heart Governor is closely associated with the Heart, and one of its functions is to protect the Heart. The Triple Heater includes the three heaters or burning places where heat and Energy are produced: the thorax, solar plexus and the lower abdomen.

ZANG	FU
Lungs • Intake of Ki from air • Combining Ki from air with Ki from food to nourish the whole body • Mental vitality and positivity	**Large Intestine** • Receives food from the Small Intestine, absorbs wanted fluids and excretes unwanted matter in the stools • Ability to 'let go'; self-confidence
Spleen • Transformation of Ki of food into Ki for the body • Gives ability to concentrate, think and analyse	**Stomach** • 'Rots and ripens' food in preparation for extraction of wanted Ki and nutrients by the Spleen, Small and Large Intestines • Nourishes intellectual thinking
Heart • Helps in formation of Blood from the Ki from food and air • Circulates the Blood, and controls the Blood Vessels • Houses the Mind, including our consciousness, thinking, feeling, and long-term memory	**Small Intestine** • Receives food from the Stomach and separates the nutritious parts from those that are not wanted which are passed on to the Large Intestine • Mental discrimination and decision-making
Kidneys • Provides fundamental Ki for all other Organs, and for birth, growth, development and reproduction • Nourishes the spine, bones and brain • Gives impetus and willpower	**Bladder** • Stores unwanted fluids and excretes them in the urine • Gives courage
Heart Governor **(Pericardium or Heart Protector)** • Protects and aids the Heart • Circulation of the Blood around the body • Influences relationships with others	**Triple Heater** **(Triple Burner)** • Distributes Ki and warmth throughout the body '•Opens emotional interactions with other people
Liver • Ensures a smooth flow of Ki to produce optimum physiological functioning and emotional stability • Creates humour, creativity and positive emotions, and the ability to plan	**Gall Bladder** • Stores bile produced by the Liver and secretes it into the Intestines • Ability to make decisions and move forwards into action

The Meridian System

The Energy system most used in Shiatsu is the system of Meridians. Each of the twelve Organs is linked with a Meridian, or channel of Energy, so that we have the Liver Meridian, Heart Meridian, and so on. Each Meridian travels partly through the body, connecting with various Organs and Chakras, and partly over the surface of the body. The Lung Meridian, for example, travels through the lungs and throat, then emerges onto the surface of the body at the front of the shoulder, and travels down the arm to end on the thumb. One end of each Meridian is inside the body, and the other end is on the hands or feet.

These twelve main Meridians are bilateral; that is, there is an identical Meridian on both sides of the body. There are two more Meridians used in Shiatsu; the Governing Vessel that runs up the centre of the back and the Conception Vessel (or Directing Vessel) that runs up the centre of the front of the body. On each Meridian there are various places which are particularly useful in changing the Energy flow in the whole Meridian. These are often called acupuncture or acupressure points, and in Shiatsu are called Tsubos. Figure 5 shows the pathway of the Meridians over the surface of the body.

Energy flows into the Meridians from the Chakras and the Organs of the body, and also from the outside into the ends of the Meridians on the hands and feet, and through the Tsubos. Each Meridian also has a short connecting pathway to two other Meridians, so that Energy flows from one Meridian to another. This Energy flows cyclically through the twelve main Meridians, as shown in Figure 6.

Working on the Meridians has a variety of effects. Firstly, because they run over the body surface and also into the body, working on the outside of the body affects the internal functioning of the Organs. The basic Shiatsu treatment that you will learn to give in Chapter 6 will help improve the Organ functioning, as well as have a beneficial effect on the hormonal system and the autonomic nervous system (this controls many body functions that automatically happen, such as movements of the intestines and bladder). With further training in Shiatsu, treatments can help alleviate a wide range of problems within the body. How amazing to be able to help the inside of the body by working simply with your hands on the outside of the body!

HG   Heart Governor
LG   Lung
HT   Heart
KD   Kidney
LI   Liver
SP   Spleen
CV   Conception Vessel
GB   Gall Bladder
ST   Stomach

Direction of Energy

Fig. 5 The Meridian System Front View

LI   Large Intestine
TH   Triple Heater
SI   Small Intestine
BL   Bladder
GB   Gall Bladder
GV   Governing Vessel

Fig. 5 The Meridian System Back View

Secondly, the flow of Energy in the Meridians over the surface of the body affects the skin, muscles and joints. Therefore many problems on the body surface can be aided with Shiatsu, such as headaches, tension in muscles, and backaches. Shiatsu is one of the most effective remedies for this kind of problem.

Thirdly, the flow of Energy through the Meridians also affects our moods, emotions and thinking. So Shiatsu often helps lift negative mental states and remove prevalent undesirable emotions and moods. One of the beautiful things about working with Energy is that it affects a person's physical, mental and spiritual state. As these different aspects of us are all composed of Energy, any change in Energy flow will have an effect at all levels of our being. Different people may be more aware of the benefits of a Shiatsu treatment at one or another level.

The different Energy systems in the human being are all interconnected, so working on one Energy system will also affect all the others. So with Shiatsu working on the Meridian system, changes will also happen in the Chakras and subtle bodies.

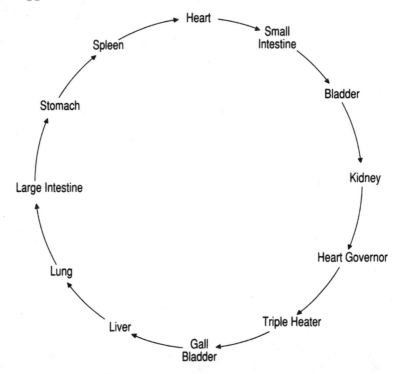

Fig. 6 The Cyclic Movement of Energy Through the Meridians

Tsubos

The flow of Energy in the Meridians can be affected by giving pressure or other stimuli anywhere along the length of a Meridian travelling over the surface of the body. However, certain points on the Meridians have been found to be commonly most effective in changing the Energy flow in the Meridians, and so have the greatest beneficial effect in restoring health. These are the approximately 365 points used for the insertion of needles in acupuncture.

In acupuncture and acupressure, only this limited number of points is used. In Shiatsu the whole length of a Meridian is worked on and not just the acupuncture points. As well as using some of the acupuncture points, any point that feels imbalanced is held to affect the Energy at that point. In Shiatsu it is considered that there are an unlimited number of Tsubos, which can be found anywhere on the body. Chapter 11 will tell you how to find many of the commonly used points and the kinds of problems that they can be useful for. This chapter is placed towards the end of the book as you will find it much easier to locate and use Tsubos after Our Energetic Constitution developing your sensitivity to Ki through practising full-body Shiatsu for a while.

An Energetic Definition of Health

As we are working with Energy, we need to be able to define health in Energetic terms. An Energetic definition of physical, mental and spiritual health could be:

1 Having an approximately even distribution of Energy in all the Meridians and other Energy systems; that is, the amount of Energy in all parts of the body is balanced.

Based on Figure 6 on page 26 showing the Energy flow through the twelve Meridians, this can be illustrated as:

When there is much more or less Energy in a Meridian or part of the body, physical and psychological symptoms arise. It never ceases to amaze me that when someone points out an area of pain, there is always an imbalance of Energy there (either too much or too little) and that simply redressing the balance causes the pain to disappear.

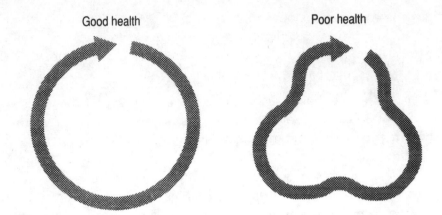

Good health   Poor health

Fig. 7

2 Energy is flowing, rather than being blocked or trapped. Life is Energy in movement. When Energy stops moving, then we become less alive, and our health is reduced. This can be illustrated as shown:

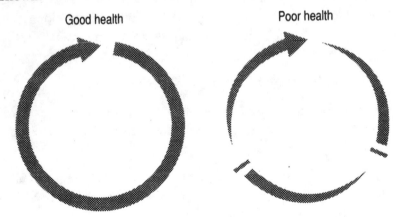

Good health   Poor health

Fig. 8

3 Having a strong flow of Energy.
The more Energy we have within us, the greater our physical vitality and stamina, mental positivity and clarity, and the wider and deeper our consciousness.

This definition of health may seem impossible to attain. This is true! We are used to a static definition of health, such as, 'the absence of any obvious symptoms or signs of illness'. With such a definition, either we are healthy or we are not. The above Energetic definition of health recognizes that health is relative; that is, we can always improve our health. It is open-ended, and allows for us continually to increase our physical, mental and spiritual health.

Working with energy

From the Energetic definition of health, it is easy to see what we are trying to do in giving Shiatsu. We want to:

1 Rebalance the Energy in different Meridians and areas of the body – reducing the Energy where there is too much, and increasing the Energy where there is too little.

2 Where Energy has become stuck or blocked, get it moving.

3 Increase the total Energy within a person. It is only possible to do this in a limited way by giving Shiatsu. The main ways of increasing our Energy are through our daily way of life, such as our choice of diet, full breathing, sufficient physical exercise and a positive mental attitude. However, during the Shiatsu treatment described in this book a person becomes deeply relaxed, and in this state stops using up Energy and receives more from the outside. With regular Shiatsu a person can learn to maintain a more relaxed state all the time. They will then not waste their Energy in unnecessary tension, and can continually receive more Energy from the outside.

When you begin giving Shiatsu, you may not be able to detect your friend's Energy clearly, so you will probably not feel where Energy is high or low or blocked. However, if you carefully follow the directions in this book, especially the Basic Principles, you will be working on a person's Energy and you will automatically tend to rebalance their Energy and clear Energy blockages. Those receiving your Shiatsu will certainly feel the difference! With practice, areas of high and low Energy will begin to reveal themselves to you.

CHAPTER 3

Exercises to Perceive Ki

Here are a few exercises to enable you to feel Ki, so that it becomes more real for you. Most people who try these exercises for the first time can feel Ki. If you cannot, do not worry! It does not mean that you never will be able to, as everybody can learn to perceive Ki with a little practice. For all these exercises it helps if you are feeling calm and relaxed, and are in a quiet environment without distractions. For the second and third exercises you will need a partner.

Exercise 1: Feeling Ki Between Your Hands

Stand with your feet about shoulder width apart and stretch your hands above your head. Now rub them together vigorously so that they become really warm and alive. Then also rub the backs of the hands and your wrists and forearms. Drop your hands to your sides, then shake them, throwing your hands away from you as if you were throwing water off your hands. Stretch your hands up above your head and repeat the rubbing, followed by the shaking. Now hold your hands out in front of you – they will feel warm and alive, due to the extra blood and Ki flow that you have generated in them.

Drop your hands to your sides, take a deep breath and relax your body as you breathe out. Repeat this two or three times. Hold your hands about 3 feet apart with the palms facing each other, relax, and let your mind become empty. Now focus your attention on the space between your hands and slowly move the hands towards each other. Keep your awareness on any feelings between your hands. If your hands get very close, do not let them touch; take them back out to 3 feet apart and start again.

When your hands get within 6 or 12 inches of each other you will probably feel some kind of sensation, such as warmth or tingling in your hands, or the feeling that you have an invisible bouncy balloon between your hands. This is the point at which the etheric aura of the two hands meet; the rubbing and shaking of the hands generated a stronger Energy field around your hands.

Take your hands out to 3 feet again and repeat the exercise until the feeling becomes more definite. When you get to the point of a definite feeling between your hands, play with it, moving your hands in and out slightly. Many people find their first sensation of Ki exciting!

Fig. 9 Feeling Ki Between Your Hands

Exercise 2: Feeling Ki Around Another Person

Now we are going to repeat Exercise 1, but feeling the Ki around another person. Ask your partner to sit on a straight chair or on the floor. You are going to feel the etheric aura around their head and shoulders, as it is usually strongest and so easiest to feel here. Repeat the rubbing and shaking of your hands – the more Ki in your hands, the more sensitive you will be to perceiving Ki. Take a few deep breaths and relax your body and mind as you breathe out. Now take one hand 2 or 3 feet to the side and above your partner's head, and slowly move your hand towards it. Focus your awareness on the space around their head. If you get very close, take your hand back out to 2 feet and start again.

You will probably get a similar sensation as in Exercise 1 when you get 2 to 6 inches from the head. When you perceive their aura, move your hand in and out a little so as to feel repeatedly the boundary of the aura. Then you can work around the head and down over the shoulders, moving your hand out and in a little to keep feeling the aura. Keep going until the sensation becomes quite definite.

If you have difficulty feeling the aura, it is usually because the mind is too busy with thoughts. Relax yourself and let it settle down, then try the exercise again.

Fig. 10 Feeling Ki Around Another Person

Exercise 3: Directing Ki With The Mind

This exercise is a little different, but is interesting as it shows how we can control the Ki flow in our bodies to some extent with our minds. Get your partner to stand in front of you with their feet shoulder width apart. Put your arms around their hips and pick them up off the floor so that you can gauge their weight. Keep your back straight and bend your knees to make the lift to protect your own back. (Ideally choose a partner approximately the same weight as you. If you have back problems that may be aggravated by lifting, you had better not attempt this exercise.)

Now tell your partner to bend their knees very slightly (this automatically drops their Ki downwards into their abdomen) and to lean backwards a little so that they have more weight on their heels than on the balls of their feet (this encourages the flow of Ki down the back of the body). They should also look down towards the ground, and stay serious, as laughter or even a smile brings Energy upwards in the body. Then they can imagine themselves becoming very heavy, as heavy as lead. They can imagine Energy flowing down through their head, through their body, down their legs, and into the ground, making them heavier and rooted to the ground.

This visualization can be repeated for one or two minutes. Then, with your partner continuing their visualization, pick them up again. The difference in weight is generally obvious; often the partner is almost impossible to get off the ground!

Now try the opposite, getting your partner to stand up straight, looking upwards with a smile, and with their weight tipped slightly forwards so that there is more weight on the balls of their feet than on their heels. They should imagine Energy flowing upwards from the ground into their feet, up through their legs, up the body and out of the top of their head. This should be continued for one or two minutes, so that they feel as light as a feather. Then, with your partner continuing the visualization, put your arms around their hips again and pick them up. Generally they will seem to fly into the air. Watch their head on the ceiling!

In this exercise you will feel how much your partner can change their weight by directing their Energy with their mind. The better their concentration, the bigger the difference you will feel in their weight

Fig. 11 Lifting a Partner

when they make themselves heavy and light. You can swap around and try making yourself heavy and light for your partner to feel. Unfortunately for those who feel that they are overweight, visualizing being lighter does not alter the reading on weighing scales! A mechanical instrument does not register the difference in weight, only a human lifter who uses Ki to lift with. If you have spent time with children, you may have already noticed how a child that does not want to be picked up can make themselves feel very heavy. Some martial arts masters who are very practised in controlling their Ki can make themselves so heavy and rooted that even four people cannot pick them up.

Hopefully these three exercises have made the world of Ki more real to you. When giving Shiatsu, variations in the amount of Energy in different areas of the body and in different Meridians and Tsubos can be clearly felt. Unfortunately this can be difficult at first because one is touching the receiver's body, and the physical sensation of touching tends to dominate the sensing of Ki. With practice in giving Shiatsu, everyone can learn to feel the Ki too.

PART 2

Learning to Give Shiatsu

CHAPTER 4

Practical Details

Preparations for Giving Shiatsu

Shiatsu has the great advantage of needing no equipment, so you can give Shiatsu almost anywhere, at any time. However, the following guidelines for ideal preparations and environment will enable you to give better Shiatsu and for the receiver to benefit more from treatment.

1 The ideal clothing for both the giver and receiver is a single layer of loose cotton clothing, such as a track or jogging suit, or a T-shirt and a loose pair of thin cotton trousers (not jeans!). Ki does not flow easily through artificial fibres, so if they are worn by the receiver it will be more difficult for you to make contact with their Ki. If you wear artificial fibres, your Ki cannot flow so easily, making your Shiatsu less effective.

It is also advisable to wear natural fibres – cotton, wool, silk or flax – for normal daily wear to allow your Energy to move more freely around the body and between your body and the environment. Remember, life is Energy, so if you constrict or cut down on the Energy you receive, you will feel less alive. This is more important for clothing worn directly against the skin, such as underwear, stockings, trousers or shirts.

For Shiatsu, the clothing must also be loose to allow you to move freely and for you to be able to move the receiver's body freely when giving stretches.

2 The room where you are giving Shiatsu should be quite warm, as the receiver usually cools down a lot as they relax. If it is warm enough, you will probably want to be wearing only light clothing yourself. If you think the room may be a little cool, have a blanket handy, and while you are giving Shiatsu to the upper body you can cover the lower body, and vice versa.

3 Unlike some forms of massage, Shiatsu is ideally given with the receiver lying on a mat on the floor. This allows you to use your weight effortlessly to give Shiatsu, rather than your muscular strength. The mat needs to be soft enough to make the receiver comfortable, but also firm so that the weight given on the body does not get taken up by the mat instead of affecting the receiver. Two to four blankets, folded in half if necessary, with a clean sheet over them are good to begin with. A Japanese futon (a thin all-cotton mattress) one to three layers thick is ideal.

4 The room must give enough space for the receiver to lie down, and for you to be able to move freely all around them. This means 3 or 4 feet at their head and feet and their sides.

5 The room should be clean and tidy. Looking at this Energetically, dust and dirt are stores of stagnant Ki that will subtly block the Ki flow of the giver and receiver. If belongings are chaotically or messily left around the room, their chaotic Ki will subtly interfere with your concentration and focus during the Shiatsu. A clean, orderly room allows your Ki to move clearly. This of course applies to your daily living space as much as it does to the place you prepare for giving Shiatsu.

6 Have one or two cushions handy in case your friend is uncomfortable lying on the mat. For example, when lying face down with the head turned to the left or right, some people's necks become stiff or painful. Often they do not realize until they come to turn over onto their back, when there is a shriek of pain! To prevent this put a cushion under one shoulder and tell them to turn their head towards it. The cushion could also be put under the upper chest.

If people have stiffness in the knees, cushions can be placed under the lower legs. Sometimes when people lie on their back a small cushion is needed under the lower back to prevent pain.

7 The room should be as quiet as possible. Noise tends to distract you and can prevent the receiver relaxing fully. You may need to take a telephone off the hook, and to put a 'do not disturb' notice up on the door. Some people like to play some quiet, relaxing music while giving Shiatsu.

8 Make sure your fingernails are cut short. You do not want to give acupuncture instead of Shiatsu! Long nails can be quite painful for the receiver.

9 Do anything else you can think of to increase the comfort and relaxation of the receiver, and your own ease of movement and concentration.

When Not to Give Shiatsu

There are some situations when it is advisable not to give Shiatsu.

1 If you or the receiver have had a large, heavy meal, wait several hours before giving Shiatsu. The Ki in the body will be directed inwards for the digestion of the food, so less Ki will be circulating around the body in the Meridians, making the giving or receiving of Shiatsu less effective. It is fine to give or receive Shiatsu after eating lightly.

2 Don't give pressure on recently broken bones, varicose veins, deep cuts, or other injuries. The receiver probably won't appreciate your resetting their fracture!

3 Shiatsu can be very helpful during pregnancy, especially for relieving the back pains that often arise. However, there are certain areas on the body that give strong stimulation to the womb. Shiatsu on these places can be useful during labour to stimulate stronger contractions, but should not be used during pregnancy. These areas are:
  (a) The ankles. In fact, it is safest not to give any heavy pressure to the feet or legs below the knees.
  (b) The fleshy area on the hands between the thumb and the base of the first finger.
  (c) The top of the shoulders just either side of the neck.
  (d) The abdomen.

4 If someone has been rushing about or is feeling very emotional, give them a little time to calm down before giving them Shiatsu. Directing them to take some long, deep breaths will help them to calm down more quickly.

In addition, people with certain problems or conditions who may be helped by an experienced Shiatsu practitioner should not be treated by someone just beginning to learn Shiatsu.

5 Do not give Shiatsu for at least several weeks after a person has had an operation, or after a woman has given birth.

6 Avoid giving Shiatsu to people with serious health problems such as cancer, multiple sclerosis, severe arthritis, heart problems, and so on. Shiatsu can be very helpful for these people, but a precise diagnosis and treatment is needed. People with serious health problems are often very low in overall Ki, with big imbalances between different areas and Meridians. An inaccurate Shiatsu could deplete them of Energy, or worsen symptoms. You could try just doing their hands and feet.

There may also be people who do not have any obvious symptoms or named illness, but who appear to you to be looking ill. These people may well be building up big health problems which haven't yet surfaced to create definite symptoms. If you feel uneasy about giving such a person Shiatsu, follow your intuition.

Remember, before you give anyone Shiatsu, ask them if they have any health problems, and if they are pregnant. And if you are in any doubt about whether or not you should give them Shiatsu, don't.

Possible Effects of Your Shiatsu Treatment

Most people will feel relaxed and rejuvenated after your Shiatsu. Beneficial effects may be noticed days or even weeks later, so make a point of always asking people a few days after the Shiatsu if they have noticed any changes. This is very useful feedback for you. Commonly reported changes include feeling more relaxed, sleeping better, being more flexible with the release of areas of tension, feeling lighter and more alive, the disappearance of minor problems like backache or tired eyes, or that a weight has been lifted from them.

A few people may experience changes that do not seem so welcome. It will help you to know of the most common reactions, and the probable causes.

1 *Tiredness* Many people will take five or ten minutes to come out of their deep relaxation, and be ready to take on the world again. This is natural. However, a few people feel exhausted, and want to do nothing but have a long sleep. These are generally people who keep going on 'nervous tension', which is actually tension in the body. When Shiatsu removes the tension, a state of underlying tiredness or need to rest is revealed. You can advise these people to rest or sleep until they feel recuperated. Unfortunately this is not always possible with the hectic pace of modern life.

2 *Coughing, mucus or colds* During or after the Shiatsu a person may begin coughing or producing mucus from the nose. Rarely, this may turn into a cold. Here the body has been stimulated to discharge some of the excess fats, sugars and other foods eaten in the form of mucus. As practically everyone in modern society has a good deal of excess in their bodies, the discharge of some of this excess is a welcome event.

Sometimes when mucus is present, a cold virus is able to infect the body, giving symptoms like aching, tiredness and coldness. It should be realized, though, that the cold virus is not so much the cause of the problem as the result. Only when body cells are in a less healthy state will they be susceptible to infection by a virus. So if somebody starts discharging mucus or develops a cold after receiving Shiatsu, you can explain that this is beneficial for their health!

3 *Headaches, other aches and pains* Occasionally a person will develop a headache or aches or pains in other parts of their body after Shiatsu. Generally they last no longer than twenty-four hours. There are two common causes of this. Firstly, Shiatsu can release Ki that has been locked up in areas of tension for a long time. When this Ki is released, it can surge around the body until it settles down to a new balance. While the Ki is surging, an excess or deficiency of Ki may temporarily occur in a part of the body, causing an ache or pain. You can reassure the person that the pain is part of a process of the body moving to a state of greater balance and health.

A second common cause of pain is that you have worked too hard or too long on a particular part of the body. The ideal amount of pressure to give to the body varies widely between different people. You can imagine that a small, frail elderly person would need a lot less pressure than a large, muscular young adult. In the exercises of the next chapter you will learn how to gauge how much pressure to give, so that this is unlikely to happen.

A particular case is someone who regularly has headaches or migraines. It can be tempting to spend longer or to give more pressure on the head in an effort to help them. However, this can bring on a headache by bringing more Ki to the head where there is already an excess. It is more important to relax the shoulders and neck, and give Shiatsu to the whole body. Even without touching the head, these people can be helped by full-body Shiatsu rebalancing Ki in the whole body.

If a headache or pain persists for longer than two or three days, it would be advisable for the person to seek guidance from a qualified Shiatsu practitioner or other health professional.

4 *Release of emotions* Every area of tension or weakness in the body is associated with certain held emotions, feelings and thoughts. When a person's Ki is stimulated to move and rebalance, they may experience these feelings. Often they may relate to some event in the past when the person experienced a strong emotion, but instead of expressing it or resolving it inwardly, they suppressed it. During the Shiatsu it is generally beneficial for people to express any strong feelings or emotions that come up, so that they can be dealt with for good. A little gentle encouragement from you can be a lot of help in this. Some people may want a good cry, and can be given some warm comfort.

5 *Feeling nothing at all* Occasionally, when asked, a person will say that they haven't felt any effects at all from your Shiatsu. This can be very discouraging when you are just beginning to learn. However, don't be put off! This comment usually says more about the person than about your Shiatsu. Many people are quite 'disconnected' from their bodies, with little awareness of areas of tension, weakness or other sensation. Only when they experience strong pain do they realize that something is wrong. So they will be unlikely to register the effects of your Shiatsu consciously, even though it may have been beneficial. Shiatsu can be a useful way of helping these people to become more in touch with their bodies. Encourage them to be more aware of your touch and the effects it has.

One cause of this insensitivity is eating a typical modern diet, high in animal fats. As the body cannot use up all of the fat, it accumulates in and around the organs of the body, and also under the skin. These fat deposits act as a great insulator to Ki, blocking its flow. Shiatsu is generally less effective for people with much fat accumulation, as it is more difficult to get the body's Ki flowing. You may have to work with as much weight as you can, still to be told by the receiver that they can't feel anything!

If someone experiences these or other seemingly unwelcome effects from your Shiatsu, explain to them the probable causes of their symptoms. This can make them feel a lot happier about Shiatsu, rather than being left with a bad impression.

CHAPTER 5

Preliminary Exercises

In learning the practical side of giving Shiatsu, this is a very important chapter. By practising these exercises you will learn how to use your Ki to affect a receiver's Ki. In the next chapter we will look at the techniques used in giving Shiatsu. For these outward techniques to be effective, it is important that you are using your Ki and not just performing them physically.

During these exercises you will be introduced to some Basic Principles for giving Shiatsu. When you are following these Basic Principles you will be primarily using your Ki rather than your physical power, and you will automatically primarily affect the receiver's Ki rather than their physical body. So even though you may not yet be sensitive to your friend's Ki, you will be moving and balancing it. Good reports from those receiving your Shiatsu will be evidence of this.

Exercise 1: Abdominal Breathing

We have three main centres in the body, as shown in Figure 12. The **abdominal centre** relates to the lower three Chakras and is concerned with our individual existence on Earth. When there is a lot of Energy in the abdominal centre we feel centred and grounded, confident, calm and peaceful, with plenty of physical vitality.

The **heart centre** is related to the heart and throat Chakras, and is concerned with our relations to other people, to nature, and the outside world. When this area is active we feel more love, empathy and compassion for people.

The **head centre** relates to the brow Chakra and to mental activity. This may be more intellectual, analytical thinking or more imaginative and intuitive thinking.

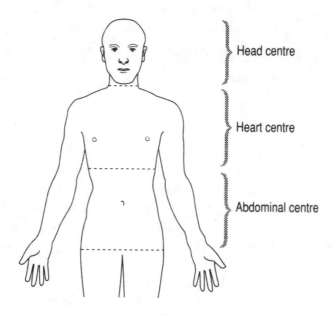

Fig. 12 The Three Main Centres of the Body

When we are physically active our Energy moves into the abdominal centre. When we are interacting with other people in an open-hearted way, Energy moves more to the heart centre. When we are thinking a lot, Energy gathers in our head. (Thinking too much or for too long can create a headache caused by an excess of Energy in the head.)

Ideally, our Energy should be approximately evenly distributed between these three centres, giving a balance with the practical, social and mental aspects of life all fulfilled. However, this is often not the case. Due to differences in diet, activity, education, social norms and other factors, particular centres may be over or underactive. Some people are 'all in their heads', others are 'all heart', and some are 'doers' without much thought or heart.

Different cultures often have broadly different Energy distributions (this partly accounts for the difficulty that is often experienced in communication between different cultures). Modern Western culture puts a lot of emphasis on mental development, whereas Far Eastern cultures traditionally put greater emphasis on developing centredness and groundedness. People from tropical and subtropical countries are often much more emotional and open about their feelings than people living in colder climates.

Shiatsu, coming from Japan, puts greater emphasis on the abdominal centre which is called the *Hara*. This is a very useful practice for us generally head-centred Westerners, and is one of the great benefits of learning Shiatsu. Here we are going to use our breath to change our Energy distribution in our body. When we breathe in, we take in not only oxygen but also Ki from the air. The air and oxygen are taken into our lungs, but with our minds we can direct the Ki to any part of the body we choose to strengthen the Ki in that area. With abdominal breathing we direct this Ki to the Hara, to increase our centredness, groundedness and vitality.

Abdominal breathing is ideally practised just before giving a Shiatsu treatment. However, if you practise it for five minutes a day, say after getting up in the morning, for a period of one to two months, your Energy can permanently become more centred in the Hara. This will make you feel more grounded with more vitality during your normal daily activities, which can make a real difference to your experience of daily life. And once you have got the hang of the exercise, you can practise it at almost any time; standing in a bus queue, sitting at work, while washing up, or when driving a car. Any time you feel flustered, tired or uptight, it can help you become calm and centred in dealing with the daily challenges of life.

The Exercise

For this exercise you need to sit with a straight back, to maximize the Ki taken into the spiritual channel. If you can, sit in *seiza*, the traditional Japanese way of sitting, as shown in the following illustration. However if this position is uncomfortable, sit cross-legged with a cushion under your bottom, or on a straight-backed chair. Put your hands together in your lap. Take a few deep breaths and relax your body and mind as you breathe out. We will now build up to the full exercise in stages.

Fig. 13 Sitting in Seiza

Stage 1

Place one hand on your chest and the other on your abdomen below the navel. You are now going to breathe with just your abdomen, and not with the chest. Take a slow breath in, keeping your chest still and allowing your abdomen to expand. Then relax, letting the air out with your abdomen falling inwards. Repeat this breathing for two or three minutes, then take a rest and practise it again. Breathe as deeply as you can while keeping the chest still, by expanding the abdomen as much as possible. It feels a bit like blowing a balloon up as far as it will go.

Some people find abdominal breathing quite easy straight away; for others it can be a difficult exercise. One reason for this is that in modern culture we are unconsciously taught to breathe more superficially using only the chest. (This makes our perceptions, thinking and living more superficial, compared with also using our abdomen which makes us more rooted, with deeper and wider perceptions and thinking. If you watch babies breathing, they mostly use their abdomens.) Another reason for difficulty in practising abdominal breathing is tension in the diaphragm, the sheet of muscle at the bottom of the rib cage separating the lungs from the abdominal organs, or general stiffness in the liver, stomach, intestines, and other organs in the abdomen.

Practise stage 1 until it is easy for you and you can do it with your hands in your lap instead of on your chest and abdomen. Then progress to stage 2.

Stage 2

Place the palm of one hand over the area below your navel, and the other hand on top of the first hand. Take a slow breath in through the nose and visualize the air travelling down through your body to the Hara beneath your hands. You may like to close your eyes to aid concentration on the visualization.

Hold your breath for three or four seconds, keeping your attention on the Ki gathered in your Hara. Then slowly let the air trickle out of your mouth (you lose less of the Ki breathing out of the mouth in this way than if you breathed out of the nose). Repeat this breathing for two or three minutes, visualizing the Ki travelling down to your Hara with each in breath.

Slowly open your eyes, look around, and observe how you feel. Different? Practise abdominal breathing regularly, and these effects will become a more permanent part of your being.

Fig. 14 Breathing Ki into the Hara

Exercise 2: Centred Movement on the Floor

Abdominal breathing helps to centre our Ki in the Hara. Now we are going to practise moving from this centre, so that we use our Ki to give Shiatsu rather than our physical, muscular strength. When we use our Ki to give Shiatsu, we primarily affect the Ki of the receiver. Also, after giving Shiatsu, rather than feeling tired from exertion, we feel uplifted and energized from the increased Ki flow in ourselves. This is one of the great rewards of giving Shiatsu; we get as much from it as the receiver!

The Exercise

Get down on your hands and knees. Have your hands and knees about shoulder width apart, with your arms either straight or almost straight, whichever is most comfortable. Relax! Let your body flop as much as possible while holding this position. Check that you are not tensing your shoulders, back, neck or arms. You are now giving perfect Shiatsu to the floor!

Fig. 15 'Standing' on all Fours

Notice that this is effortless – you are not pushing on the floor, just resting your weight on it. And there is no need for any tension in your body. You are now experiencing the first three Basic Principles of giving Shiatsu:

1 Use your weight, and not your strength.

2 Give Shiatsu effortlessly.

3 Stay relaxed; don't tense up.

This may seem strange to you, as we are so used to making efforts to achieve various aims or goals in our lives. What you are learning through this exercise, and will learn further through giving Shiatsu, is that life need not be a constant struggle, requiring endless effort and strain. The whole of life can become an easy flow from one activity to the next.

Now let's practise moving. Rock your weight forwards a little so that you are putting more weight on the floor through your hands. Now slowly rock your weight more onto your left hand, then your left hand and knee, then both knees, then your right knee, and onto your right knee and hand, then onto the right hand, and finally back to both hands.

To make these movements you will have been moving your whole body, with the movement centred on your Hara. Make another half dozen or so slow circles, then do the same number in the opposite direction, moving clockwise rather than anti-clockwise. Then come back to the central all-fours position.

While you are moving, observe yourself following the first three Basic Principles, using your weight effortlessly and without tension. Furthermore, notice that to change the weight you are giving to the floor through your hands, you move your whole body, and that your body's centre of gravity is in the abdomen. You are experiencing the fourth Basic Principle:

4 Change your weight on the receiver by moving your whole body, with your Hara as the centre of movement.

Now rock your body forwards to increase the weight your hands are giving to the floor, hold the position for four or five seconds, then rock backwards with more weight on your knees. Rock forwards onto your hands again, hold for four or five seconds, then rock back. Repeat this about a dozen times, observing how, with your whole body movement, you increase and decrease the weight you are giving to the floor through your hands. Then come back to the central position. You have now been following two more of the Basic Principles:

5 **Use your weight at right-angles to the body surface (in this exercise, the floor).**

6 **Hold your weight on the receiver for a short time.**

The reason for always using your weight at right-angles to the body surface is that you then contact the body's Ki. Coming in at an oblique angle, you will have much less effect on a person's Ki flow. As the body is rounded, unlike the floor, you will need to adjust your position so that you are always effortlessly using your weight at right-angles to the receiver's body surface.

When you are leaning your weight on a person or giving a stretch, the position is held for a short time, usually between five and fifteen seconds. This is because the movement of increasing your weight on a person has a more physical effect, but while you hold still, Ki moves within the receiver. While holding a position, there is a particular moment when the place you are holding or stretching 'opens', and a lot of Energy moves at once. The time taken for this opening to happen is usually between three and twenty seconds. If you don't hold, this opening and movement of Energy never happens.

It is unlikely that you will feel this opening phenomenon when you first practise Shiatsu, so I advise that you generally hold all movements for four or five seconds.

Exercise 3: Centred Movement on a Partner

Now we are going to practise applying the Basic Principles while giving Shiatsu to another person instead of the floor! Ask your partner to lie down on their front on a mat or several blankets. Move their left arm away from their body so it lies approximately at right-angles to their body, then kneel on their left side facing at right-angles to the line of their body. Take up the all-fours position as before, with your right hand on the hard sacrum between their hips and your left hand between their shoulder blades. You should feel exactly the same as when you were on all fours on the floor – relaxed, with arms straight or just slightly bent, resting your weight on them effortlessly. (It is amazing how at this point the mind can start thinking, 'I must do something now', and one starts tensing up and using muscular effort!)

Fig. 16 'Standing' on all Fours on a Partner

Rock your weight back a little onto your knees, then forwards onto your hands, and hold for four or five seconds. Then rock back onto your knees, then forwards again and hold. Repeat this simple movement about a dozen times, checking that you are:

1. using your weight and not your strength;
2. moving effortlessly;
3. staying relaxed;
4. moving your whole body;
5. giving your weight at right-angles to your partner's back;
6. holding your weight for four or five seconds each time you lean forwards.

Also, ask your partner if you are using too little or too much weight. If you are using too little, the Shiatsu can feel ineffective. To increase the weight on your hands, move your body further forwards over their body. If your partner is large, muscular, or in good health, you may need to move your knees back further away from them so that you can give more weight through your hands.

If you are using too much weight, your partner will say it hurts! Generally one does not want to cause pain when giving Shiatsu, as it makes the receiver tense up and this tension prevents their Ki flowing. So ease up and use a little less weight; that is, don't move your body so far forwards onto your hands.

When students first practise this exercise, they often give too little weight. It can be quite surprising just how much weight you can use when you are in this relaxed state. So keep asking your partner for feedback, and experiment with using different amounts of weight to find the middle point between being ineffectual and causing pain or discomfort. At this middle point you will be giving Shiatsu most effectively.

This middle point will obviously vary a lot with different people. Generally larger, more muscular, fitter and younger adults need more weight, and with smaller, frailer, less fit and older adults or children, less weight is needed. However, the best thing to do at first is to ask the person what feels right for them. This is more accurate than guessing!

When you find the middle point in this exercise, you can then lean your weight onto your partner confidently. This is very important, because if you are hesitating or holding back for fear of hurting them, you will also be withholding your Ki. This makes the Shiatsu less effective. This is just the same as any action in life – if we do something 'whole-heartedly' and with 'body and soul', we not only enjoy ourselves more but also achieve far more. So find the right weight for your partner, and then lean your weight on them with body, heart and soul!

The middle point or right amount of weight will obviously be different for each part of the body. Large structures like the back, thighs and bottom usually need a lot of weight, and smaller and softer structures like the ankles, hands, abdomen and face need less. So the first few times you practise the full-body Shiatsu treatment described in the next chapter, you will probably need to keep asking your partner if you are using too little or too much weight. This may seem to break into the flow of the Shiatsu, but is well worth doing at first so that you quickly learn to make your Shiatsu as effective as possible. With time you will develop the sensitivity to know how much weight to use for a particular person and part of the body.

That's enough on weight! Now rock forwards and backwards a few more times, ensuring that you are giving equal weight on both hands. Don't be biased towards either hand. You are now experiencing another Basic Principle; that when using two hands to give Shiatsu:

7 Use equal weight on both hands.

Having practised your own movement, we are now going to progress to moving your hands over the receiver. The right hand will stay in the same place on the sacrum while the left hand moves down the back, giving Shiatsu to the large muscles lying either side of the spine. Put the heel of your left hand about 1½ inches to the right of the spine, between the shoulder blades. Let the palm and fingers rest on the back. Now rock your body forwards, giving equal weight through your right hand and heel of your left hand, hold for four or five seconds, then rock backwards.

Fig. 17 Palming Down the Back

Move your left hand down the back about a hand's width, rock forwards and hold, then rock back. Move your left hand down another hand's width, and continue down the back until your left hand reaches the hip. (This movement of your hand down a part of the body is called 'palming'.)

Take your left hand back up to the level of the shoulder blades and repeat the Shiatsu down the right side of the receiver's back. If you are unsure about how much weight to use, ask your partner how it feels.

Having worked down the right side twice, place the heel of your left hand about 1½ inches to the left of the spine between the shoulder blades. Give Shiatsu to the left side of the spine twice as you did for the right side.

Your partner should now be feeling wonderful! From practising this first Shiatsu form, you can appreciate another Basic Principle:

8 Move with a steady rhythm throughout your Shiatsu treatment.

Besides the specific effects of the various forms used in a Shiatsu treatment, the rhythm of your movement has a big effect. If you slow up and spend too long working on one area, your Ki flow and that of the receiver tend to slow up, and you will not be so effective in getting their Energy moving. If you go too quickly the receiver will probably not relax, and without proper holding the Shiatsu will only have a superficial effect. Between these two extremes is a comfortable, natural rhythm and effortless flow, rather like the feeling of rocking a baby. This will make the receiver feel very nurtured and open to your loving touch.

There is one more Basic Principle, which applies to the overall Shiatsu treatment:

9 Keep in contact with the receiver throughout the Shiatsu.

When you are moving your own body around the receiver to give Shiatsu to different areas, you may take both hands off them for several seconds. Try to avoid this. While you are moving yourself, keep one hand lightly on the receiver's body. You may need to slide a hand from one area to the next to keep in contact. When a person becomes deeply relaxed during a Shiatsu session, prolonged loss of contact can give a slightly unpleasant feeling of being deserted. You do not have to be fanatical about this – a second's loss of contact will not matter, but five or ten seconds will.

If you have incorporated the Basic Principles into your treatment, you will already be giving fine Shiatsu. If you are still a little unsure about using them, go through the exercises in this chapter again. Here are the Basic Principles for you to refer to.

The Basic Principles for Giving Shiatsu

1 Use your weight, and not your strength.

2 Give Shiatsu effortlessly.

3 Stay relaxed; don't tense up.

4 Change your weight on the receiver by moving your whole body, with your Hara as the centre of the movement.

5 Use your weight at right-angles to the body surface.

6 Hold your weight for a short time.

7 Use equal weight on both hands.

8 Move with a steady rhythm throughout your Shiatsu.

9 Keep in contact with the receiver throughout your Shiatsu.

CHAPTER 6

A Basic Shiatsu Sequence

Now that you have practised how to give Shiatsu, we can look at some techniques. In this chapter a number of basic techniques are described to make up a full-body Shiatsu treatment. There are hundreds of different possible techniques and those presented here are a selection of those most commonly used. Once you have become proficient in using these, you can learn more from other books or by attending courses.

Before you begin, remember the following points.

1 Don't forget to ask the receiver if they have any health problems, as described in Chapter 4, to check if it is OK for you to give them Shiatsu.

2 Try to follow the directions on different techniques exactly. In each technique you should feel comfortable and relaxed. If the position feels awkward or difficult to maintain, try shifting your position around until you feel comfortable. Only when you are relaxed will your Ki flow and will your Shiatsu be effective.

3 When you are leaning your weight on the receiver or giving a stretch, hold the position for three to five seconds. As you practise this full-body Shiatsu treatment, you may sometimes feel that you want to hold for a longer time in certain areas. Follow this intuition, and hold for as long as you feel appropriate.

4 Each technique can be performed once or several times. To begin with, do each technique once unless the directions state otherwise. Again, as you practise, you may sometimes feel like repeating a technique – follow your intuition.

5 When you are giving pressure on the receiver's back, abdomen or chest, you should increase the pressure while they breathe out, and then reduce the pressure long enough for them to breathe in. If you can't see the breathing, then tell them when to breathe in and out. It helps if you breathe with them. You will probably find that you naturally begin to breathe out whenever you lean your weight or move into a technique, synchronizing your breathing with all your movements.

6 It is difficult to describe how much weight you should use when giving Shiatsu. Generally, if you are relaxed and not using force, you will probably be able to use more weight than you might think. With practice, you will develop the feel for the right pressure for a certain place on the body of a particular person. However, at first it can be difficult to judge, so ask the receiver for feedback: 'Is this too hard?', 'Am I using enough weight?', or simply, 'How does this feel?'.

7 With a little practice, this full-body treatment should last about forty to fifty minutes. It may take you a little longer at first. However, if you continue to take over an hour to complete it, you are probably going too slowly, and not keeping up a good rhythm.

The Back and Shoulders

1 Begin by kneeling on the left side of the receiver, who should be lying face down. Put your right hand on the sacrum, and pause for a few seconds while you become calm and centred. 'Tune in' to the person's body, emotions, thoughts and breathing.

Fig. 18

2 Keeping your hand on the sacrum, palm down the far side of the back twice, and then down the near side twice. Begin between the shoulder blades and continue down to the small of the back.

Fig. 19

3 Step across the receiver, and position their arms with the palm upwards and the elbows slightly bent. Put the palm of your left hand between the spine and shoulder blade, and with the other hand palm twice down the whole length of their right arm and onto the palm of the hand. You may well feel tension in the shoulder relax as you work down the arm. Now repeat this on the other arm.

Fig. 20a

Fig. 20b

4 Place your thumbs close to the spine between the shoulders. Steady your thumbs by giving firm pressure with your fingers also. Lean your weight forwards and hold for a few seconds. Move your thumbs down an inch and repeat. Continue down the back, and then on to the bony sacrum.

Fig. 21

5 Bring one arm up gently over the back, and hold in place at the elbow with your knee or foot. Pull the shoulder up as you lean your weight downwards through your fingers, pressing under the shoulder blade. Repeat several times, working your fingers under the bottom and top of the shoulder blade.

Fig. 22a　　　　　　　　　　　　　**Fig. 22b**

6 Release the arm, hold onto the wrist and raise the arm. Turn the arm so that the little finger points towards their head – this locks the elbow. Hold the shoulder firmly with the other hand and rotate the arm in little circles to loosen the shoulder. Then move the arm towards the receiver's head until you feel some resistance, and hold this stretch for a few seconds. *Be gentle*! It is easy to go too far and cause pain. Rotate the arm a few times and repeat the stretch. Place the arm on the floor and repeat stages 5 and 6 on the other arm.

Fig. 23

The Buttocks

7 Move down to the receiver's hips, and with one hand on the sacrum, palm one buttock. Start at the top of the buttock and work down to the top of the leg.

Fig. 24

8 Keep the same hand on the sacrum, and use your thumb to press three or four points down a line through the centre of the buttock.

9 Put your other hand on the sacrum and repeat stages 7 and 8 on the other buttock.

Fig. 25

The Legs

10 Bring your leg back so that you are kneeling beside the receiver. With your left hand on the sacrum, palm down one leg from the top to the ankle, moving your hand down about a palm's width each time. Quite a lot of weight can be given on the legs, but only light pressure can be used on and just above and below the knee otherwise you will hurt the front of the knee. If the receiver has long legs or if you have short arms, you may need to move the hand on the sacrum down to the upper leg.

Fig. 26   a   b

11 Put your moving hand on the heel, and lean forwards to stretch the inside of the lower leg.

Fig. 27

12 Repeat 10 and 11 on the other leg.

13 Move to between the receiver's legs, and with one hand on the sacrum, raise the lower leg towards the buttocks, holding onto the foot. Lean your weight onto both hands, giving a good stretch to the front of the thigh and lower leg. Remember to hold for a few seconds. If the foot easily reaches the bottom, the receiver won't be getting much of a stretch, so move the foot to the outside of the bottom.

Fig. 28   a

14 Bring the leg back so that the lower leg is vertical. Place one hand on the ball of the foot, and lean most of your weight onto it to stretch the Achilles tendon. Place the foot back on the floor.

Fig. 29

15 Repeat stages 13 and 14 on the other leg. You should hardly have to shift your own position while doing these stretches on the legs.

Turning Over

Now ask your friend to turn over, slowly. They will probably be quite relaxed by now, so you don't want them to jump up suddenly and disturb this relaxation.

The Feet

16 Kneel at the feet and, taking one foot, hold onto the back of the heel and press your thumb along three lines on the sole of the foot, holding each position for a few seconds.

Fig. 30

Fig. 31

17 Stretch open the top of the foot by pressing down with the heels of your hands and pressing up with your fingers. This releases tension held in the top of the foot.

Fig. 32

18 Stretch the toes upwards, and then downwards (carefully, as some people's toes don't stretch downwards very far). Repeat a few times to stretch the top and bottom of the foot.

Fig. 33a

Fig. 33b

19 Hold onto the foot firmly with one hand, and hold the base of the little toe firmly between your thumb and first finger. Rotate the toe to loosen its joint with the foot, then lean back and stretch the toe away from the leg. You may get a crack as stagnant Energy is released. Do the same for all the other toes.

Fig. 34

20 Repeat stages 16, 17, 18 and 19 on the other foot.

The Hips and Legs

21 Move to the left side of the receiver, place one hand on the abdomen, and with the other hand palm down the front of the leg from the top to the ankle. Repeat on the other leg.

Fig. 35   a   b

22 Move to between the receiver's legs, put one hand on the abdomen, and raise one leg with your other hand under the knee. Place the foot on the floor and slide your hand to the front of the knee. Raise the leg off the floor and bring the knee towards the receiver's chest. Rotate the leg, going up the inside of the body and then bringing it outwards away from the body, and down into the next rotation. Move your whole body to rotate the leg, don't just use your arm.

Fig. 36

23 Lean on the leg, bringing the knee towards the chest, to stretch the buttock and back of the thigh. Place the foot back on the floor, slide your hand back under the knee, lift the leg and place it down on the floor again. Be careful not to let the leg drop suddenly as this could hurt the knee.

Fig. 37

24 Repeat stages 22 and 23 with the other leg.

The Abdomen

25 Move to a position at right-angles to the receiver's side and place both hands across the abdomen. Push into the abdomen with the heels of your hands, then pull into the abdomen with your fingers, somewhat like kneading bread. Do this ten or fifteen times.

26 Now kneel with your thigh against the receiver's. Rest your left arm on your leg and push up with the left hand under the abdomen. Use your right hand to palm in a circle around the abdomen twice, pressing twelve times at the positions of the twelve hours of a clock.

Fig. 38   a   b

Fig 39

Fig 40

Now repeat, using your fingers to press more deeply. This gives deep massage to the organs of the abdomen: the stomach, small and large intestines, liver, gall bladder, pancreas and spleen. Some places may be sensitive so go gently at first.

Fig 41

27 Put your right hand on the lower abdomen below the navel, push in gently and hold for ten or twenty seconds to bring Ki into the receiver's Hara.

Fig 42

The Chest

28 Move to the receiver's head and kneel with your knees either side of their head. All the rest of the Shiatsu treatment is given from this position.

Bring each arm out to the side with the palm upwards to open the shoulder. Put the heels of your hands inside the shoulder, and lean your weight onto the shoulders. Hold for a few seconds, rock backwards, and then repeat a few more times. You may well feel the shoulders moving towards the floor as the chest opens.

Fig 43

29 Keep one hand on the shoulder, and place the other hand on the lower ribs on the opposite side of the body. Lean forwards onto both hands, stretching the chest open. Shift your moving hand up towards the head a little and repeat. For a man, you can continue to move your hand up, pressing in five or six places until the moving hand reaches the shoulder. For a woman, pressure on the breasts is uncomfortable so bring your hand inside the breast, using the side of your hand to give pressure.

30 When your moving hand reaches the shoulder, keep it there and use your other hand to repeat stage 29 on the other side of the chest. You may well notice that the receiver's chest is now broader and more open, and that the shoulders naturally lie closer to the ground.

Fig 44a

Fig. 44b

The Arms and Hands

31 With one hand on the shoulder, palm down the length of the arm and onto the hand twice. Give lighter pressure on the elbow.

Fig. 45

32 Pick up the hand, and holding the hand and wrist, lean backwards to stretch the arm and shoulder. Hold the stretch for a few seconds, release, then stretch again.

Fig. 46

33 Open the palm of the hand by pressing down with the heels of your hands and upwards with your fingers. Repeat three or four times.

Fig. 47

34 Use one thumb to press down three lines on the palm.

Fig. 48

Fig. 49

35 Grasp the hand firmly with one hand, and hold the base of the little finger with your other thumb and first finger. As with the toes, firmly rotate the finger to loosen its joint with the hand.

Fig. 50

36 Squeeze the base of the little finger, move your fingers up a little and squeeze again. Work up to the tip of the little finger.

Fig. 51

37 Repeat stages 35 and 36 with the other fingers and thumb.

38 Put the hand down on the floor and repeat stages 31 to 37 on the other arm and hand.

The Neck

Most people carry a lot of tension in the neck and will really enjoy Shiatsu in this area. Promoting Ki flow in the neck can help relaxation and Ki flow in the whole body.

39 Place the fingers of one hand on the spine just below the skull and put the fingers of your other hand over the first hand's fingers. Raise the neck slightly so that the head tips backwards a little. Lean backwards to stretch the neck away from the body, with your fingers pulling on the back of the skull. Hold for a few seconds, release, then repeat. If there isn't too much tension in the neck, you will feel it lengthen, maybe by half an inch or so.

Fig. 52

40 Place your hands on the sides of the head with your fingers behind the ears and your thumbs in front of the ears. Pick up the head, turn it to the side, and put it down on one hand. This hand supports the head while you work on the neck with the other hand.

Use your thumb to press into the top of the neck just under the back edge of the skull. Begin just behind the ear, move half an inch towards the spine and press again. Continue until you reach the spine, where you will find a depression between the top vertebrae and the skull. Press into this depression.

Fig. 53   **Fig. 54**

41 Palm the side of the head, beginning at the front and pressing in three or four places to cover the whole side of the head.

42 Put your moving hand back on the side of the head with your fingers behind the ears, pick up the head and turn it to the other side. Repeat stages 40 and 41 on the other side of the neck and head. Put your moving hand back on the side of the head, pick the head up and place it gently back down on the ground.

43 Put one hand under the neck and slide it under the head. Hold the neck with the other hand, and using both hands stretch the head to the side. Hold for a few seconds, then return the head to the floor. Slide your other hand under the head and do the stretch for the other side of the neck.

Fig. 55a

Fig. 55b

44 Slide one hand under the head again, pick it up, and place your forearm behind the head with the hand on the opposite shoulder. Bring your body up so that your forearm brings the head up, stretching open the back of the neck. Hold for a few seconds, then withdraw your forearm and gently replace the head on the floor.

The receiver must be fully confident that you have full control of their head and won't drop it! If there is any doubt, they will tense their neck, and your Shiatsu will have less effect.

Fig. 56

45 Stretch the neck as in stage 39 again. The neck will often stretch more this time as your other work has relaxed the neck.

The Head and Face

46 Grip the head gently but firmly with one hand and use the thumb of the other hand to press in a line from between the eyebrows to the top of the head, moving about half an inch each time.

Fig. 57a

Fig. 57b

47 Rest the fingers firmly on the sides of the head and use your thumbs to press in two lines from the inner edge of the eyebrows to the top of the head.

Fig. 58

48 Keep your fingers firmly on the sides of the head and use both thumbs to work from the inner edge of the eyebrows across the forehead above the eyebrows to the temples.

Fig. 59

49 Now use your thumbs to work along the bony ridge under the eyes, moving about a quarter of an inch each time.

Fig. 60

50 Press just to the side of the nostrils, then move in a line under the cheekbones.

Fig. 61

51 Press with one thumb between the nose and upper lip, and then with both thumbs out across the upper jaw.

Fig. 62a   **Fig. 62b**

52 Press with one thumb just below the lower lip, and then with both thumbs out across the lower jaw.

Fig. 63

53 Place the fingers of both hands under the lower jaw and lean back to give pressure on the underside of the jaw.

Fig. 64

54 You have now finished your Shiatsu treatment. Place your hands lightly on either side of the head for ten or fifteen seconds, then slowly draw your hands away. Tell the receiver that you have finished, and that they should lie quietly for a few minutes until they feel ready to get up. Move to their side and sit quietly until they get up. They may well want to ask you some questions, or to share their experience of the Shiatsu with you. You may also want to ask them how the treatment felt to get some useful feedback.

Fig. 65

Congratulations! You have probably just completed your first full Shiatsu treatment. You may well be feeling that it was very complicated, and that there is an awful lot to remember. Now is the time to get some more practice in. Run through the basic Shiatsu sequence with some more friends over the next few days or weeks. You will be surprised at how easily you will remember all the actions once you have run through the full sequence a few times.

Learning to give a basic Shiatsu treatment is rather like learning to ride a bicycle. At first you have to concentrate hard on all your movements, but once you get the hang of it you can stop thinking about the bicycle and concentrate on cycling along the road. You can start experimenting to find out just what you can do on the bicycle, as well as how to avoid cars! After giving a dozen or so Shiatsu treatments you will be able to stop thinking about yourself and concentrate on the receiver. Then, as with riding a bicycle, Shiatsu becomes much more interesting, for you will begin noticing just how different everyone's bodies are, and how the body actually asks you to vary your Shiatsu for different individuals and for different areas on one body.

The next chapter will give you some guidelines on how to adapt your Shiatsu to different individuals' needs. The following three chapters will expand your understanding of the Energetic basis of life, and will enable you to further develop and refine your Shiatsu treatments.

PART 3

Developing Your Shiatsu Further

CHAPTER 7

Adapting Your Shiatsu for Different People

Now that you have mastered the basic Shiatsu sequence, you can concentrate more on how to vary your Shiatsu for people of different ages, characters and levels of health.

You already make your own intuitive judgements about people's health and character. You can now learn to incorporate this judgement into your Shiatsu treatments. It can be so important to get the general approach to the whole person right. You can give a technically brilliant Shiatsu treatment to someone but unless your overall approach is appropriate it could be completely wasted. So remember, you can ask people you are giving Shiatsu to, 'How does this feel?' 'Is this too hard or too soft?', and so on.

Also remember that in Chapter 3, you did an exercise by picking up a partner who first thought of themselves as being heavy, and then as light. You will have felt a difference in their weight merely because of their different thoughts, because we can move Energy with our minds. So in giving Shiatsu, if we are holding the thought in our mind that we want to give a sensitive, supportive, strong or vigorous treatment, this will make a difference to the quality of the Shiatsu we give.

A few examples of what you may perceive about people, and how to adapt your Shiatsu to their individual needs, are given overleaf. As you give Shiatsu to more and more people you will develop your ability to adjust your approach for each person.

The Receiver	Your Treatment
Overall, the person's energy seems weak, with a lack of vitality, possibly with a limp body and a lack of mental positivity	Firm, supportive, nourishing Shiatsu
Overall, the person's energy seems full, with an excessive amount of physical and maybe emotional energy	A calming and relaxing Shiatsu
An emotionally sensitive person	A gentle, sensitive Shiatsu, with care not to give too much pressure which could make them withdraw fearfully
A large, physically strong person	Use more of your weight to give stronger pressure and stretches
A small, frail, elderly person	Go very gently, taking care not to use too much pressure or to stretch too strongly
A healthy and active ten-year-old child	Use less pressure than with an adult, and if the child is restless, give a shorter treatment
Low pain threshold	Go gently!
High pain threshold, or enjoys feeling some mild pain	Go more strongly

CHAPTER 8

The Next Step – Kyo and Jitsu

The next step in developing your Shiatsu is to start using Kyo and Jitsu. In Shiatsu we are primarily working with Energy. Obviously the amount or intensity of Energy in different people and in different parts of the body is very basic to this approach. Kyo and Jitsu are used to describe the states of deficient or low Energy (*Kyo*) and excess or high Energy (*Jitsu*).

Kyo and Jitsu can be used at different levels, considering the amount of Energy in a whole person, in different areas of the body, in the Meridians, and at specific Tsubos.

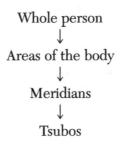

Students beginning to learn Shiatsu generally find it easier to diagnose Kyo and Jitsu on the broader levels of the whole person and in areas of the body. As you study Shiatsu further, you will progress to perceiving Meridians and Tsubos through touch and visually, and will then be able to diagnose Kyo and Jitsu in the Meridians and Tsubos.

Diagnosis of Kyo and Jitsu

It is relatively easy to tell whether the whole person is more Kyo or Jitsu. If someone is low in physical energy, with a rather limp-looking body without much muscle tone, and maybe a rather negative or depressed emotional or mental expression, they could be said to be more Kyo. They will probably give the feeling of needing support and nourishment. So the overall direction of your Shiatsu needs to be firm, supportive and energizing. A person who is lively, active and expressive with high muscle tone could be described as being more Jitsu. They may give the feeling of needing to stop and relax for once. So you can make your Shiatsu more calming and relaxing, for example by going slowly without sudden movements.

Kyo and Jitsu also exist in different areas of the body. In Chapter 2 we saw that our life and health depend on the flow of Energy through the body, and that ideally Energy should be more or less evenly distributed in different Chakras, Organs and Meridians. Nobody ever achieves a perfect balance, but we can all work to improve the balance of Energy. One way of doing this is through Shiatsu. As you become more practised in giving Shiatsu, you begin to pick up on areas of the body where the Energy is low or high.

Kyo and Jitsu can be diagnosed visually by looking at a person, from touching a person during a Shiatsu treatment, and by the receiver's response to your touch. Before giving a Shiatsu you may see imbalances, which give a general guide as to which parts of the body need some extra attention. Then during the Shiatsu, through your touch you will pick up on Kyo and Jitsu areas in greater detail. Also while giving Shiatsu, if you are perceptive about how the person is feeling, you can pick up on their response. Of course they may also tell you how your Shiatsu feels. So giving Shiatsu is quite a curious blend of both diagnosis and treatment.

Visually, if you quickly scan your eyes over another person, your attention will be drawn to certain places. These areas are usually those which are out of balance. The body could be described as consisting of 'mountains' where areas stand out, due to an excess of Ki, and 'valleys' where areas appear hollow or weak, because of a deficiency of Ki. If a person is in relatively good health, there are relatively few mountains and valleys, and these are not so marked. If the valleys and mountains are more marked, then the person's Ki is more imbalanced and their health is probably poorer.

	Kyo	Jitsu
Visual Diagnosis	Area is hollow or depressed	Area is raised, standing out
	Weak looking with a lack of muscle tension	Excess muscle tension
Touch Diagnosis	Feels unnaturally soft (or surface tension with weakness beneath)	Feels hard
	May feel cold	May feel hot
	Feels empty or lifeless	Feels full and alive
	Feels needy, asking to be held	Feels repelling, not wanting to be touched
	Difficult to find, hidden	Usually easy to find, obvious
Receiver's Response	Feels vulnerable	Feels safe
	Deep, unpleasant pain	Local discomfort or pain
	Deep relaxation and nourishment	Local relaxation and relief

As you become more practised in giving Shiatsu you will probably naturally begin noticing that some parts of your friends' bodies feel hard and tense, while other areas feel soft, with a lack of muscle tone and an empty or lifeless feeling. These are physical signs that the areas are Jitsu or Kyo. When a place is greatly depleted in Energy (that is, very Kyo) a stiff surface tension may develop, hiding the underlying Kyo. As you give Shiatsu to such an area, the surface tension will usually relax, revealing the weakness below. At some point in your learning of Shiatsu you will also come to sense Ki directly, as in the first two exercises you practised in Chapter 3. As this sense of Ki becomes more definite it can be used as the main way of diagnosing Kyo and Jitsu during your Shiatsu.

Thirdly, Kyo and Jitsu can be identified by the sensations of the person receiving your Shiatsu. Kyo places are weak, and therefore vulnerable. If pressure is given too suddenly or too hard, a person experiences deep unpleasant pain and feels invaded or attacked. Their body may recoil to protect this place of weakness. On the other hand, if gentle, sensitive, firm and supportive pressure is given, the person relaxes deeply, and feels great relief and nourishment from the Shiatsu. Appropriate Shiatsu on Kyo areas, Meridians or Tsubos brings deep relaxation and healing to the whole person.

If too much pressure is given on a Jitsu place, it may feel uncomfortable, but only in that localized area and not throughout the body. It is more bearable than too much pressure on a Kyo place. Appropriate Shiatsu on Jitsu places creates relaxation more at the surface and at just that location, and does not have such a deep or wide effect as Shiatsu on a Kyo place.

Treating Kyo and Jitsu

From what has been said above, you can see that varying your Shiatsu according to Kyo and Jitsu will increase the effectiveness of your treatment. When you follow the basic Shiatsu sequence described in the last chapter, you will actually tend to rebalance both Kyo and Jitsu areas. However, as you become more conscious of Kyo and Jitsu within the body, your Shiatsu can become more specific, and so more beneficial.

Some general guidelines can be given on how to vary your Shiatsu according to Kyo and Jitsu. These are not rigid rules, but just pointers to help you develop your own sense of what is appropriate for different people and different parts of the body.

Kyo	Jitsu
A sensitive touch is needed	Use pressure with the palms or thumbs for a shorter time to move the excess Energy out of the area
Hold pressure with the palm or thumb for a longer time, for ten or fifteen seconds or until you feel the place has come alive.	
	Stretching for a short time can be very effective at moving the Energy out of Jitsu areas
Stretches can be held for longer to bring Energy into an area.	
	Movements like rocking and shaking parts of the body can help move excess Energy out of an area

Don't get too intellectual in using Kyo and Jitsu; for example, getting in a panic because you can't identify Kyo and Jitsu areas in a particular person. Rather, as you 'tune into' the bodies of the people you are giving Shiatsu to, Kyo and Jitsu will 'appear' to you. You can then change your approach according to what you see or feel, either holding a Kyo area or Tsubo longer, or working to dispel the Energy from a Jitsu area or Tsubo.

When beginning to look for Kyo and Jitsu within the body, Jitsu places often stand out more than Kyo places. It can then be tempting to work more on these Jitsu places, trying to dispel the excess tension and Energy. However, this way of working will only have a more superficial effect, unless Kyo places are also identified and treated appropriately. It is generally most effective to work on both Kyo and Jitsu places within a full-body Shiatsu treatment, and not just concentrate on either one of these imbalances.

If someone has pain in a particular part of their body, the Energy in that place is always either Kyo or Jitsu. Pain caused by an area being Kyo is generally of the chronic, nagging, dull, deep kind, whereas Jitsu pain is usually more acute, intense or stabbing. If you can rebalance the Energy in painful areas, the pain will almost always go. If the person has had the pain for a long time, then several treatments may be needed to rebalance the Energy and remove the pain.

It takes many Shiatsu treatments to really get the hang of perceiving and working with Kyo and Jitsu. It is a gradual process of learning to perceive Ki more clearly. Regular practice is the key to a better understanding, as in learning any practical skill. So now that you are gaining in confidence in giving healing Shiatsu treatments, find some more friends or willing members of your family to keep practising on.

CHAPTER 9

The Energetics of Food

Oriental medicine uses several approaches to balance Energy in the body, and so promote health or alleviate illness. Having examined one approach, Shiatsu, we are going to look briefly at another: the use of diet. As well as giving Shiatsu treatments, Shiatsu practitioners frequently give clients advice on steps that they can take themselves to promote their health, such as advising changes in diet and activity, and practising specific exercises. These life style changes complement Shiatsu treatment very well, and can greatly add to the health benefits. As with other aspects of Oriental medicine, food is considered mainly in Energetic terms.

At present, the common way of looking at food is based on the scientific analysis of its constituents – carbohydrates, fats, protein, vitamins, minerals and fibre. This approach is useful in ensuring that we get enough of the various nutrients that our bodies need, and that we do not overconsume certain nutrients like fats or simple sugars. However, this modern nutritional theory alone does not ensure good health; one may be eating enough of the necessary nutrients and still get ill. It also gives little indication of the emotional, psychological and spiritual effects of different foods.

Our understanding of the relationship between food and health can be greatly extended by looking at the Energetic qualities of the foods we eat. Just as the body has traditionally been regarded Energetically, food can also be understood in terms of Energy. One can then understand how foods interact and change the Energetic constitution of the body. It can give an exact method of comprehending the effects of particular foods on us physically, emotionally, mentally and spiritually.

Furthermore, a knowledge of the Energetic nature of the body and of foods combined with methods of Oriental diagnosis of ascertaining the condition of the various Organs and systems of the body enables one to work out exactly which foods are most harmful and most beneficial for a particular individual. This approach can be used by anyone to improve their health and steadily reduce the chances of their suffering from illness in the future, as well as for alleviating a very wide range of health problems.

This chapter gives a brief introduction to the Energetics of foods and their effects on our health, with broad recommendations on how to eat a healthier diet. The next chapter, on Oriental diagnosis, will give you a more precise idea of how particular foods may have contributed to health problems, and of beneficial dietary changes that can be made to alleviate them.

Yin and Yang

In considering food as Energy, we need a way of describing Energy. The most useful way is to use Yin and Yang, which describe the direction of the movement of Energy. (This is different from Kyo and Jitsu, which describe the intensity of Energy.) Traditionally it was considered that the two fundamental directions of movement are expansion and contraction, and that the interplay between these two create all forms and events in nature and the universe. Therefore everything can be described in terms of Yin and Yang.

This may seem very simplistic, and in a way it is, but its simplicity is its strength. Using Yin and Yang can help us see the essential or most basic qualities of life. Also, as everything can be described in terms of Yin and Yang, we can understand the interrelationship of any two aspects of life or nature, such as the influence of our food on our physical health, moods and emotions and spiritual awareness, how we can adjust our food when living in different climates or seasons, and according to particular kinds of activity.

Yin is used to describe any phenomenon where the Energy is expanding:*

Fig. 66

Yang is used to describe any phenomenon where the Energy is contracting:

Fig. 67

We use many pairs of opposite qualities to describe and understand our lives – hot and cold, day and night, male and female, extrovert and introvert, rich and poor, happy and sad, young and old, to name a few. The table overleaf gives some other examples of Yin and Yang.

---

* Here I have used the definitions found in macrobiotic teachings, as most books dealing with the Energetic qualities of food are from this source. George Ohsawa, who began teaching macrobiotics, changed the traditional view that Yang is expansion and Yin is contraction to Yang symbolizing contraction and Yin symbolizing expansion, thinking that this system would be more easily understood by people in the West. This was the only change he made; other qualities such as hot and cold, night and day, and active and passive remained the same as in the traditional definition.

This change of definition should present no great problem for students of Oriental philosophy and medicine. The words 'Yin' and 'Yang' are quite arbitrary – different words could be used, or the classification of Yin phenomena and Yang phenomena could be reversed. The only important thing, as with all language, is that their basic definition is clearly stated so that a word can carry meaning to another person. However Yin and Yang are defined, the universal symmetry of nature remains unchanged and eternal.

	Yang	Yin
Movement	Contraction	Expansion
Natural Cycles	Day	Night
	Summer	Winter
	Activity	Rest
	Work	Play
	Tension	Relaxation
	Growth	Decay
	Life	Death
Air	Carbon dioxide	Oxygen
	Hotter	Colder
	Dryer	Wetter
	Positive ions	Negative ions
Vibrations	Longer waves	Shorter waves
	Red – Orange – Yellow – Green – Blue – Violet	
	Radio waves	X-rays
The Body	Male sex	Female sex
	Solid organs, e.g. liver	Hollow organs, e.g. stomach
	Parasympathetic nervous system	Sympathetic nervous system
	Inbreath	Outbreath
	Physical and social activity	Mental and spiritual activity
Dimension	Time	Space

The Yin and Yang of Food

When we look at our food in terms of Yin and Yang, the most fundamental division we can make is between animal and plant foods. Using
the pairs of qualities given above, we can work out whether animals or
plants are more Yin or Yang. Animals are active, contain red blood, are
often warm-blooded, and are concentrated in that they eat many times
their body weight to create their bodies. The Energetic nature of
animals can therefore be said to be Yang. Plants, on the other hand, are
passive, are based on the colour green of chlorophyll, and are generally
cool. Plants have a more expanded form, with many leaves and numer-
ous roots in the soil, whereas the bodies of animals are compact with
their 'leaves' internally in the lungs and their 'roots' along the length of
the intestines. Plants have a more expansive, or Yin, Energetic nature.

We can also distinguish a third major category of foods. Many foods are created from various extracts from plants, such as sugar, oil, stimulants like coffee and tea, spices, and alcohol. These extracts are nearly always a more Yin or expansive part of the plants, so this group of foods is more expansive or Yin than the plants they come from.

We now have three broad groups of foods, as shown below:

Yang Foods	Balanced Foods	Yin Foods
Meat	Cereal grains	Oil
Eggs	Vegetables	Fruit juices
Poultry	Beans	Sugar
Fish	Seeds	Honey
Seafood	Nuts	Stimulants
Cheese	Temperate fruits	Alcohol
Salt	Sea vegetables	Milk
Miso		Yoghurt
		Cream
		Spices
		Most drugs, e.g. aspirin, cortisone
		Refined foods
		Most chemical food additives
		Tropical fruits and vegetables

Salt is not a living food but a mineral, and is very contractive, and so it is placed in the Yang category.

Milk has a more expansive nature. The Energetic nature of foods made from milk varies according to how they are made; hard cheeses are harder and more condensed, and are generally quite salty, and so are more Yang. Yoghurt and cream are lighter and have a more expansive Energy than milk.

Foods that grow in a hotter tropical climate (Yang) are generally more expanded or Yin. Tropical fruits like oranges, pineapples and dates and vegetables of a tropical origin, including potatoes, tomatoes, peppers and aubergines, therefore fall into the Yin category.

As we have seen, everything in our lives is created by Yin and Yang. These two forces nourish and sustain our whole being – the body, emotions, mind and spirit. At a physical level the balance between Yin and Yang has a very profound effect on our health, such as the all-important sodium-potassium and acid-alkaline balance of the blood and body, the production of hormones with opposite effects such as insulin and glycogen or oestrogen and progesterone, the expansion and contraction of organs like the heart, lungs and intestines, and in the two halves of the autonomic nervous system – the sympathetic and parasympathetic – which are basic to the smooth functioning of the entire body.

We experience the Yang force as creating inner strength and warmth, energy and vitality, tension, and the ability to be busy or working. The Yin force takes Energy outwards in the body to be used in our physical movement, actions and expression. It also has a cooling effect and creates more relaxation.

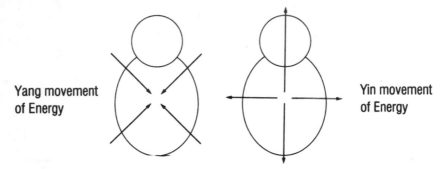

Yang movement of Energy

Yin movement of Energy

Fig. 68

Looking at this figure you can imagine how emotionally the Yang force produces more centredness, groundedness, stability, constancy and reliability, whereas the Yin force produces more expressiveness, creativity, communication and sociability.

Mentally, the Yang movement produces greater focus or concentration, more analytical and intellectual thinking, while the Yin movement produces more artistic, imaginative and creative thinking, with a broader or wholistic perspective.

When these two forces are in balance, we experience health in body and mind. In this view health can be defined as 'a balance between Yin and Yang in our physical, emotional, mental and spiritual being'. This can be illustrated as:

a balanced flow
of Energy

Fig. 69

Thinking of health in terms of Yin and Yang is also more useful as it relates to our common everyday experience. We often talk about our Energy being 'high' or 'low', being elated or depressed, inwardly turned (introverted) or outwardly turned (extroverted). Sometimes we feel 'stuck' or 'blocked' when the flow of Energy through the body is just that, and 'out of sorts' or 'off-balance' when it is imbalanced. When our Energy flow is smooth and unimpeded we feel happy, and when the Energy flow is poor we feel sadness.

A Diet of Extremes

There are many influences in our lives that affect the balance of Yin and Yang Energy within us, but our food is undoubtedly one of the most fundamental factors. We eat several times a day, day-in day-out, for all of our lives. If we look at the typical modern diet in terms of Yin and Yang we can see that it is predominantly made up of the more extreme Yin and extreme Yang foods, as shown in Figure 70. When we look at this figure it is really not surprising that in modern society we suffer from such a multitude of physical illnesses and psychological problems resulting from an imbalanced state of health.

Although people are generally eating both the extreme Yin and Yang foods, many people eat proportionately more of the Yang foods, or more of the Yin foods. Therefore problems can be caused by one of three ways of imbalanced eating – predominantly extreme Yang foods, extreme Yin foods, or a combination of both. The Energy movement in each case is illustrated in Figure 71:

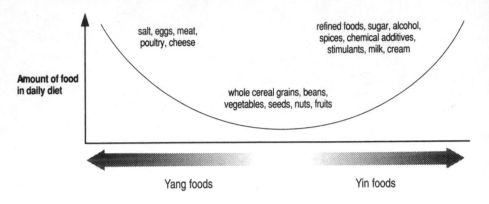

salt, eggs, meat, poultry, cheese

refined foods, sugar, alcohol, spices, chemical additives, stimulants, milk, cream

Amount of food in daily diet

whole cereal grains, beans, vegetables, seeds, nuts, fruits

Yang foods

Yin foods

Fig. 70

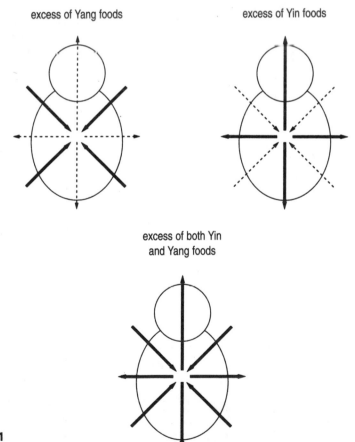

excess of Yang foods

excess of Yin foods

excess of both Yin and Yang foods

Fig. 71

In the first case when large amounts of Yang foods like meat, eggs and salt are eaten, various parts of the body become contracted, hardened and stiffened. For example, a diet high in animal fats is well known to create arteriosclerosis in which the walls of the arteries become thickened and hardened.

It is easy to see that an excess of Yang foods will cause a build-up of Energy deep inside the body. This is experienced as deep tension and the feeling of being bottled up. These people can appear 'uptight', and often keep a tight control over their emotions and life, repressing their feelings and reacting to situations logically and intellectually. The bottled-up Energy sometimes escapes in bursts, causing outbursts of anger, impatience and frustration. There is a tendency to become more rigid, stubborn and inflexible. Such people often hold on tightly to their views or way of life, denying the ideas of others and resisting any changes in their lives. Think of your friends and acquaintances and you will probably be able to identify some that have these characteristics.

When a person eats large amounts of the more extreme Yin foods such as sugar, sweets and other foods high in sugar, honey, spices and tropical vegetables and fruits, the body's organs become expanded, enlarged and weakened. Enlargement of the heart can cause poor circulation, and eventually heart problems. Expansion of the intestines is very common, causing irregular bowel movements with either diarrhoea or constipation, and more severe problems like colitis.

Consuming more of the extreme Yin foods moves Energy to the surface of the body. This can create a more surface tension or nervousness, anxiety, over-excitability and over-emotional behaviour. At the same time the energy deep inside the body becomes depleted, causing an inner weakness that may be expressed as fearfulness, worry, under-confidence or stress. Thinking tends to become vague or 'spaced out'. There may be difficulty in maintaining concentration in work or in any pursuit, and a tendency to give up on things before they are completed. Money and opportunities 'slip through the hands' all too easily. Again, review people you know and you will probably be able to think of some with these qualities.

A diet with approximately equal amounts of the more extreme Yin and extreme Yang foods brings about a variety of health problems involving contraction and expansion, such as formation of stones in the kidneys and gall bladder, many skin ailments, and breast cysts and tumours. This combination of both extremes also creates a mixture of the emotions and thinking described above. Often there are swings in mood from one extreme to the other, such as from fear to anger, or depression to aggression.

Traditional Diets from around the World

It is informative to look at the traditional diets of peoples from around the world because they often arrived at a relatively healthy way of eating through trial and error over hundreds or thousands of years. This way of eating sustained them over many generations. Much of this traditional wisdom has been lost in the modern world of mass-produced and convenience foods. We must be careful not to idealize any traditional way of eating as the ideal way, as most ancient cultures still suffered from illness, and were often constrained by the limited range of foods available locally. However many of today's diseases, especially of the serious degenerative illnesses like cancer, diabetes and heart disease, were absent or little known in many traditional cultures.

A brief look at traditional diets from around the world reveals a consistent pattern of eating. Broadly speaking, we can see two major dietary patterns. Firstly, peoples living in the far north of Asia and America, such as in Siberia, northern Scandinavia, Greenland and northern Canada, relied heavily on animal foods, as this was the main food source available to them. Judging by reports on the health of the Eskimos and other inhabitants of the far north, this diet was relatively healthy. In such an extreme cold climate with plenty of physical activity, a high animal fat diet seems necessary to provide the body heat and energy necessary for survival. This would be expected from using the theory of Yin and Yang – living in a colder or Yin climate, a more Yang diet is necessary to keep in balance with the environment. Unless we are living under similar conditions, this can hardly be considered a sensible way for us to eat.

The second major dietary pattern can be seen in peoples living in temperate and tropical climates. Some kind of whole cereal grain has usually formed the largest part of the diet with a smaller amount of beans. Fresh vegetables were eaten in fairly large quantities where available, mostly cooked, with some eaten raw. A little fish, dairy produce, meat, or certain fermented foods such as miso, tempeh, and shoyu soy sauce made from soya beans were used, with pickled vegetables like sauerkraut, and fermented drinks like beer and wine. This last group of animal foods and fermented foods may well have been included as a source of vitamin B_{12}, which is not generally present in fresh plant foods. Fruits were generally eaten in small quantities. This major dietary pattern is illustrated below.

Fig. 72

While many major cultures' diet followed this basic pattern, the specific types of foods used in each category varied greatly depending on the kinds of food plants that grew well locally. In India the main part of the meal was usually bread or rice, with a smaller amount of dahl made from beans or peas, a dish of cooked vegetables, and a small serving of yoghurt, fish or fowl. Often a little fruit or raw food like sprouted beans or salad greens was also added.

In China and Japan, most meals consisted of rice and cooked vegetables with smaller amounts of beans, fish, meat or fermented soya bean products. In parts of China, rice was replaced with millet or wheat.

North American Indians were mainly hunters and gatherers, but in the south agriculture was practised. Corn, cornbread or tortillas comprised the largest part of a meal, with smaller amounts of leafy green vegetables, beans and peas, and occasionally meat, dairy produce or fish.

The Middle Eastern diet was primarily based on a flat bread (pitta) and garbanzo beans (chickpeas) with some cooked vegetables and yoghurt, fish or meat.

These traditional diets still form the basic way of eating of a large part of the world's population. In northern Europe it is more difficult to discover people's traditional eating patterns, as this region has been most affected by industrialization and the development of many refined and artificial factory-made foods. However, bread made from wheat, barley or rye seems to be found everywhere with pasta or noodles prevalent in some Mediterranean countries, which probably formed by far the largest part of the diet. Various kinds of beans and peas were eaten in most areas, although this tradition has now been lost in many parts. Locally available vegetables were eaten, and some dairy produce, fish or meat formed a smaller part of the diet. In addition, fermented drinks like beer and wine seem to have been standard fare.

From this brief survey of dietary patterns, we can see that the diet of most stable groups of peoples in temperate and tropical climates have been primarily made up of foods in the Energetically balanced group. Is this a mere coincidence? With the extremely wide range of foods available, this can hardly have occurred by chance. Through simple trial and error over many generations this was probably found to be the most economical and healthy way of eating.

As we have seen, our modern way of eating is practically opposite to this traditional balanced Yin-Yang dietary pattern. When we have been raised on this modern diet of meat, dairy produce, sugar and refined grains it seems like the normal way to eat, but in view of the diets eaten by humankind over thousands of years around the world, it can be seen to be a very recent and localized experiment in eating. By all accounts, it is rather a failure! It has brought ever-increasing poor health and disease, as well as the widespread destruction of our soil and environment.

Eating a Balanced Diet

Choosing our food mainly from the Energetically balanced group will, over time, greatly enhance the creation of a balance in Energy in the different subtle bodies, Chakras, Organs and Meridians, and therefore also in the physical body. This balanced way of eating is shown below.

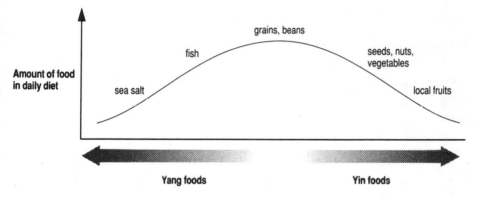

Fig. 73

For example, eating a lot of animal foods in the more Yang food group over-energizes the lower Chakras. This tends to make people more assertive and individualistic. This way of eating has actually contributed much to the whole mentality and civilization of modern Western society. When large amounts of the more Yin food group are regularly eaten, the lower Chakras become weak and the upper Chakras are over-stimulated. This can make people ungrounded and impractical, and overly preoccupied with mental and spiritual activities. Eating a diet based on the balanced group of foods will create a balance in the activity of the different Chakras, which will be reflected in greater harmony in the physical, emotional, mental and spiritual aspects of our daily lives.

Likewise, eating primarily from the balanced food group will create a chemical and Energetic balance in the blood, body fluids and cells, and in the Organs, nervous and hormonal systems. As the internal Organs of the body are intimately connected to the Meridians that pass out from them over the body, an Energetic balance in the Organs will tend to create a balanced flow of Energy in the Meridians.

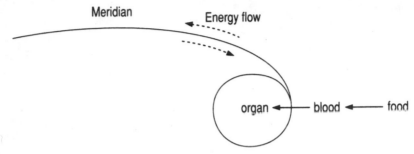

Fig. 74

To understand in more practical detail how to eat from the balanced food group, it is helpful to expand the three food groups into a more accurate continuous scale from the most Yang foods to the most Yin, as shown in Figure 75. Note that there is a good correlation between the Yin-Yang Energetic nature of foods and their sodium – potassium balance.

About 80 per cent of this balanced diet is made up of a variety of different whole cereal grains, beans and bean products like tofu and tempeh, and vegetables. Seeds, nuts, fruit and fish and/or fermented foods make up another 10 to 15 per cent. In addition, various seasonings are needed, such as a little sea salt, vegetable oil, shoyu soy sauce, vinegar, garlic, root ginger, herbs, and grain sweeteners like barley malt and rice syrup. Plus one needs some non-stimulating beverages like Three Year Twig Tea (also called Bancha or Kukicha), grain coffees like Barleycup, Caro and Yannoh, mild herb teas, or dandelion coffee. A little alcohol and fruit or vegetable juice can also be drunk.

There is not enough space in a book of this size to go into greater detail on eating a balanced diet. However, several books are given in the Further Reading Section that give much more information on the Energetic nature of foods, and how to cook balanced and varied meals.

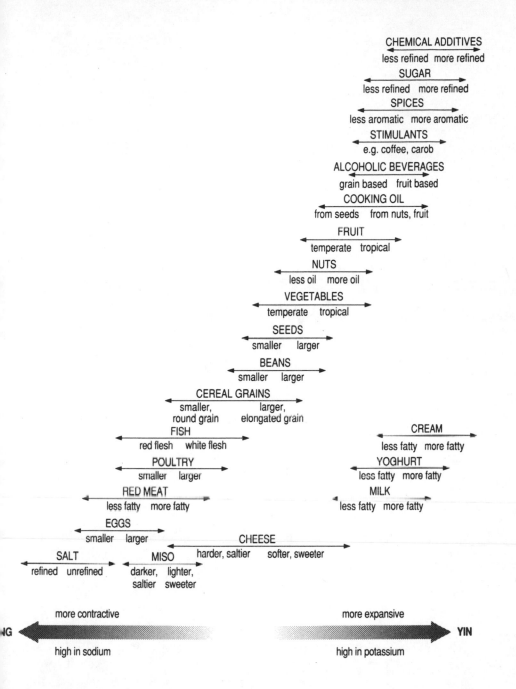

Fig. 74 Foods Arranged on a Scale From Yang to Yin

CHAPTER 10

Oriental Diagnosis and Body Reading

From practising the guidelines in Chapter 7, Adapting Your Shiatsu for Different People, you should be getting the feel of the overall direction of your Shiatsu treatments. From Chapter 8 on Kyo and Jitsu, you may now sometimes be picking up on areas of the body where a person's Ki is more imbalanced and in need of some extra Shiatsu. Chapter 9 outlined the influence that diet has on health. This chapter gives you extra information on what you can learn about a person by looking at and touching them, and how you can adapt your Shiatsu according to what you observe.

The likely dietary causes of particular imbalances and problems are also given, with guidelines on beneficial changes in diet. It should be remembered that the balanced diet plan described in the last chapter is the most fundamental way of using the Energies of food to establish Energetic balance and health in the body, and should form the basis of moves to improve one's diet.

Shiatsu and dietary changes work very well together. The Shiatsu has a more immediate effect, rebalancing and stimulating the movement of a person's Ki, while changes in eating patterns have a more long-term effect, bringing about deep changes in a person's health.

By looking at the body, we can learn a great deal about the inner health of the body and a person's emotional and mental make-up. We all actually do this intuitively when we meet and interact with other people, but very often we are quite unconscious of how we do it. For example, when we first meet someone, within a second or two we may feel drawn to or repelled by them. How we greet them and what we first say to them depends on our very rapid initial assessment of the kind of person they are. Or when we see a friend, even before speaking with them we may say, 'What's getting you down today?', or, 'What are you worried about?', or, 'You are looking happy today'.

By studying traditional methods of Oriental diagnosis and some more modern methods of body reading, we can greatly increase the amount we can learn by simply looking at a person. Many methods of diagnosis were developed in countries like China and Japan based on seeing, hearing, smelling, questioning and touching another person (or ourselves). These methods reveal much about a person's ancestors, parents and personality, their past environment and diet, and the present state of health of organs and systems within the body. In this chapter we will concentrate on postural diagnosis, in which one sees or feels imbalances in the physical structure of the body, and in the distribution of Energy over the body. These methods are of direct practical use in giving Shiatsu. Recently some Western methods of body reading have been evolved that reveal much about a person's emotional and mental make-up. This approach can be used to help people on an emotional and mental level through work on the body.

Modern Western thinking has tended to focus on the physical structure of the body such as the bones, muscles, organs, skin, and so on. As we saw in Chapter 2, we are actually multidimensional. We have a physical body and closely associated with it, the etheric Energetic body. Then there is the astral body which relates to a person's emotions, and the mental and causal bodies. All of these bodies lie over each other, although they extend outwards to different distances.

So when we look at a particular part of the physical body, say a foot, what we see is the result of what is happening in the whole of the person's physical, emotional, mental and spiritual states. This can make feet very interesting! And if someone has a problem with their feet, the main cause may be in their inner physical health, in unconstructive or Energy-blocking emotions or mental beliefs, or in impediments in their spiritual evolution.

You can demonstrate this interrelationship by standing in front of a mirror with your feet firmly on the floor, straightening your spine and neck, and bringing your shoulders back so that your back is flat. You may find that you need to take some extra deep breaths, or that your breathing deepens. You may also feel more self-esteem, stronger, more open, and thoughts may enter your mind, like how you can be more effective in your life. So by changing your physical body, other changes have happened on a physical, emotional and mental level. Shiatsu primarily affects the etheric body, and through this brings about physical, emotional and mental changes.

The Back and Front of the Body

In some people the back and front of the body appear quite different, with one stronger than the other and possibly presenting a quite different character. Physically, the back of the body particularly reflects the strength of the Energy in the Kidneys and Bladder, as these Meridians run mainly over the back. If this Energy is strong, a person usually has 'spine', that is, they have courage and initiative in standing up for themselves and for what they want or think is right. If the back appears weak, a person is likely to be weak-willed, anxious and cautious. They will probably greatly enjoy strong, supportive Shiatsu down the back of their body, giving them a greater sense of inner strength and resource. They could also reduce foods that weaken the Kidneys, especially sugar, spices, tropical fruits and vegetables, excess fluid and cold foods like ice cream, and eat more foods that strengthen the Kidneys like whole cereal grains, beans (especially aduki beans), sea vegetables, and soups seasoned with barley miso. Kidney Energy is also weakened by overwork, a lack of sleep, and an excessive amount of sex, so more sleep and rest can also help.

Emotionally and mentally, the back of the body reflects our unconscious. Very often there is a lot of tension in the back as a result of feelings and thoughts that have been pushed into the back of our minds. Frequently, releasing this tension with Shiatsu relieves people of a lot of negativity, leaving them feeling lighter and happier. Eating a lot of Yang foods like meat, eggs, cheese and salt also creates a lot of tension in the back, and therefore also contributes to the retention of old emotions and thoughts. Reducing these foods and eating a more Energetically balanced diet will help to reduce tension in the back and back of the neck.

The front of the body reflects the strength of the Energy in the Stomach, Spleen and pancreas. The Stomach and pancreas are primarily arms as a whole: heart and throat Chakras

lungs, throat Chakra

heart, circulation, heart Chakra

liver, gall bladder, spleen, stomach, pancreas, solar plexus Chakra

kidneys, bladder, small and large intestines, reproductive system, Hara, sacral and base Chakras

sexual and personal power

legs as a whole: Hara, sacral and base Chakras

stomach, pancreas, spleen

kidneys

liver, gall bladder

Fig. 76 Diagnostic Areas on the Body – Front View

liver, gall bladder

lungs, large intestine,
throat Chakra

small intestine

heart, circulation,
heart Chakra

liver, gall bladder, stomach,
pancreas, spleen, solar plexus
Chakra

small intestine, large intestine,
kidneys, sacral Chakra

bladder, reproductive system,
sexual organs, base Chakra

liver

kidneys

gall bladder

intestines, bladder, kidneys

kidneys, bladder,
reproductive system

Fig. 76 Diagnostic Areas on the Body – Back View

digestive organs, but in a wider sense the Stomach and Spleen Energy determines our appetite for food and life, and how we take in and give out on a physical, emotional and mental level. If the front of the body appears weak, a person's digestive abilities may be weak, and their appetite for life and forward movement through life may be low. Eating a lot of sweets and sweet foods frequently contributes to a weakening of the stomach and pancreas. Replacing these with naturally sweet foods like onions, parsnips, squash and dried fruits will help.

If the front of the body is strong, a person's appetite for food and for new experiences is generally strong. If there is a lot of tension in the front of the body, say in the chest, abdomen and fronts of the thighs, this appetite may be excessive. A person may then be restless, always in a hurry and busy. Relaxing this tension can help a person to become calmer.

The Top and Bottom of the Body

There is also often an imbalance between the top of the body above the waist and the bottom of the body. The strength of the abdomen, hips, legs and feet reflect our physical vitality and centredness, and the strength of our connection with the ground. If the lower body is weak while the upper body is strong, a person may be relatively ungrounded and underconfident in dealing with physical or practical aspects of their lives. However, they may be quite mentally and socially active. The Intestine and Kidney Energies are frequently weak. Spending longer giving Shiatsu to the lower back, buttocks, lower abdomen, legs and feet can help bring the person's energy down to increase their vitality and groundedness. More Yin, expansive foods like sugar, fruits, spices, coffee and chocolate bring Energy upwards in the body. Reducing these foods and eating more grains, vegetables, beans and fish will help to bring the Energy down and strengthen the Energy in the lower body. More physical exercise using the legs, such as brisk walking, jogging or cycling can also help to bring Energy downwards to strengthen the lower body.

When the lower body appears stronger than the upper body, a person often enjoys being physically active but can be 'overly grounded', without much reflection or thought about their lives. There may be a lot of stiffness and tension in the hips, legs, knees and ankles and excessive weight around the hips and thighs. If this condition has been present a long time, a person may develop osteoarthritis in the lower spine and hips. Shiatsu on the legs, and especially stretches in this part of the body, can help release this Energy so that it can move upwards to the upper body. Eating less of the more Yang, contractive foods like eggs, salt, meat and poultry and more of the balanced group of foods will also help reduce the excess of Energy in the lower body.

The Head and Neck

A common problem in modern society, present in almost everyone, is tension in the neck and back of the head, sometimes resulting in headaches or migraines. One cause of this is probably the excessive amount of time we spend in intellectual thinking. Energy moves to whichever part of the body we are using, so if we use our 'heads' much of the time, this brings a lot of Energy up into the shoulders, neck and head. Another cause relates to the Liver and Gall Bladder, as the Meridians associated with these Organs run over the back of the neck. People who eat or who have eaten a lot of meat, eggs and dairy foods, which greatly tax the Liver and Gall Bladder, generally have a lot of stiffness and tension in the back of the neck.

When the back of the neck becomes chronically tense, Energy can no longer move freely between the head and the body. Physically this can lead to headaches and problems with the eyes, ears and face. It can also trap people 'in their heads', so that they become predominantly thinkers, without their thoughts being connected to their feelings and actions which requires a flow of Energy between the head, chest and abdomen. Also, the person's thinking will tend to be rather intellectual and rigid. Shiatsu to the neck and head can release this tension, and often clears thoughts that have been persistently buzzing around a person's head, reconnecting them with their feelings. If the person is regularly eating meat, eggs and cheese, a reduction in these foods will also be of help.

When the head droops forwards, a person often has a dejected, depressed or defeated appearance. Their self-esteem and confidence may be low. Frequently the lower back is also weak, and the spine has a marked S shape. One cause of this inner collapse is weakness of the Energy in the Lungs and Large Intestine. People with this appearance commonly have problems in these organs, such as asthmas, bronchitis, constipation, diarrhoea and intestinal cramps. The Lungs and Large Intestine are especially weakened by an excess of sweet foods, such as sugar, sweets, cakes, chocolate, honey, fruit and fruit juices. There may also be past experiences which have led to dejection and a lack of belief in themselves. The chest and abdomen are generally Kyo, and more Shiatsu to these areas can help people with this drooping head posture. The balanced diet outlined in the last chapter will help to strengthen the Lungs and Large Intestine, and regular physical exercise which requires deep breathing can help in Energizing these Organs and the whole body.

The Shoulders

The shoulders also reflect the health of the Lungs and Large Intestine. The two Meridians associated with these Organs run across the top of the shoulders. Emotionally, the shoulders relate to the shouldering of responsibilities, to work and action in the world. When the shoulders are raised, giving a defensive and fearful expression, the Lung and Large Intestine Meridians are usually weak or Kyo. Shiatsu on the front, top and back of the shoulders as well as down the arms will help to strengthen the Lung and Large Intestine Energy. The likely dietary cause of weakness of the Lungs and Large Intestine are described above in 'The Head and Neck'.

In many people the shoulders are pulled forwards, curving around the upper chest as if to protect it. There is often a feeling of being weighed down by too many responsibilities or psychological burdens. Such a person is prone to feeling depressed and withdrawn, preferring to spend much of their time alone and shunning company. Again the Lungs and Large Intestine are functioning poorly, and if the whole chest is sunken the Heart and circulation may also be weak. The Lungs, Large Intestine and Heart may be too Yin or Yang, so eating the Energetically balanced diet is recommended. Breathing is often poor, so the body and brain are probably not receiving the full amount of oxygen they need. This may contribute to the mental depression and lack of Ki in the person. It is therefore very helpful to take strong regular exercise where one has to breathe deeply. This often very quickly lifts the heavy or depressed feelings. Spending too much time alone should be avoided. Sharing thoughts and feelings and having fun with other people can help in lifting the spirit and in opening the chest and shoulders.

The Back

Backs are fascinating as they reflect the condition of all the Organs of the body and the five Chakras or Energy centres governing our physical, emotional and mental disposition. Back pain is a very common problem, which is often considered to be connected only with the spine and the muscles and ligaments holding it in place. When considered Energetically, the back is a reflection of the inner health of the Organs, and of their associated Meridians.

In the physical view the causes of back pain are generally a mystery, and only symptomatic treatment is offered. With this understanding, the underlying causes of pain can usually be found, and steps taken to remedy them. With all pains, there is either an excess or deficiency of Ki in the area. By rebalancing the Ki with Shiatsu, the pain usually disappears. If the pain is long-standing or severe, changes in diet to improve the health of the organs associated with the particular area of the back may also be needed.

If there has been an imbalance in the Ki over a long period of time, the vertebrae may also be out of alignment. Adjustments to return vertebrae to their proper position may remedy this, but some people find that the vertebrae move out of place again, which is not surprising if there is still an Energetic imbalance. In these cases it can be helpful to rebalance the Energy in the area of misalignment with Shiatsu and possibly also make dietary changes. Once the Ki is balanced, the body itself will naturally tend to bring the spine into correct alignment. Adjustments will then be more successful. To understand the causes of back pain and postural imbalances, we can divide the back into four areas (see Figure 76).

The upper area is influenced by the lungs and heart, and so reflects a person's respiratory and circulatory functions. These organs are associated with our emotional expression and social nature. If this area appears weak or hollow or feels Kyo (soft, lacking in resistance), these organs and their associated Meridians are weak. The weakness may also be reflected in a weak-looking chest and drooping shoulders. The person may lack confident self-expression, and their circulation may be weak. Extra time giving Shiatsu to this area will help raise the Ki in these organs. More time on the chest and shoulders will probably be needed as well.

Sometimes the back is curved in this area, indicating that there has been a strong imbalance in Ki over a long period of time, and that the health of the lungs and heart is poorer. If the curve is great, there is a strong possibility that the person has experienced heart problems already. Shiatsu, and especially dietary changes, are needed. The organs may be either overly Yin or Yang, so a balanced diet is recommended.

The second back area reflects the organs in the centre of the body; the liver, gall bladder, stomach, spleen and kidneys. Frequently there is a lot of tension here, reflecting a build-up of Energy in this central part of the torso. There may also be problems in these organs. This area of the back also reflects the activity of the solar plexus Chakra, which is concerned with our personal power and desires, and is the seat of our emotions. If there is much tension here a person may be holding back in expressing or asserting themselves. They may be experiencing a lot of frustration, suppressed anger, or other strong emotions. Shiatsu to this area of the back and to the upper half of the abdomen can help dissipate this Energy. Often this tension is also associated with a diet high in animal products, which cause an accumulation of Ki in these organs. Reducing these foods and eating a more Energetically balanced diet could be of help.

The lower back is a common site of pain. It reflects the health of the small and large intestines, which lie in front of this area, and of the kidneys. The lower back is weak in the majority of people, because of poor health of the intestines and kidneys. It usually feels soft, lacking in resilience. When the muscles around the spine are weak, lumbar vertebrae may also become misaligned in this area, or more severely, a person may experience a 'slipped disc'. So the original cause of a slipped disc is usually poor health of the intestines and kidneys, due to an imbalanced diet and life style! The base of the spine also represents our base – our physical vitality, sexual energy and psychological groundedness. When this area is weak a person often experiences a lack of a strong root or base in their life.

During your Shiatsu, time spent holding any weak points or places which a person finds sensitive will help to strengthen the Ki in the lower back, and frequently this is enough to get rid of back pain in this area. A severe weakness in this area is generally caused by the consumption of the more Yin foods. Eating the balanced diet and taking care not to consume too much fruit, fruit juices, stimulants, alcohol and other more Yin foods can bring a long-term and permanent strengthening of the lower back and relief from any back pain in this area.

The sacrum and buttocks reflect the health of the bladder, the reproductive system and sexual organs. For example, during pregnancy, when the growing foetus puts pressure on the uterus, a woman frequently experiences pain over the sacrum. Shiatsu to the area is quite safe and can be of great help in relieving this pain. If this area appears strong, with well-rounded and firm buttocks, a person's overall vitality and sexual energy are probably strong. However, if there is tension in this area there may be excessive sexual desire, and a woman may suffer menstrual cramps. Shiatsu to disperse the Energy from the sacrum and buttocks can help diminish the cramps. Omitting animal products like meat, eggs and poultry and excess salt will also be of benefit.

If the sacrum and buttocks are weak, with a lack of muscle tension in the buttocks, the bladder and reproductive functions are probably weak. In women there may well be an erratic menstrual cycle. In giving Shiatsu, spend longer holding points over the sacrum, and work deeply into the buttocks with your palms and thumbs. This can draw more Energy into this area and strengthen the associated organs. Considering diet, weakness in the lower body is usually caused by consuming an excess of Yin foods, especially sugar. Avoiding sugar and eating a balanced diet can help strengthen this area and a person's vitality and groundedness.

The Legs

The legs and feet connect us with the ground. Energy passes from the ground into the soles of the feet and up the legs to the base and sacral Chakras and Hara. The strength of Ki in the legs reflects the strength of a person's Hara, and especially of the intestines, kidneys and reproductive organs. If the Ki of the Hara and legs is strong, a person is likely to be in touch with the practical aspects of their life, and be able to 'stand up for themselves'. However, if the Ki is weak here, the person may have difficulty dealing with the practicalities of their lives, deciding on their direction in life, and 'standing on their own feet'. They may trip up often, being unsure of their footing, both physically and figuratively. When the legs are weak a person may subconsciously stiffen or brace their legs, tensing the muscles and locking the knee joints so that they have a stiff-legged way of walking. Extra Shiatsu on the lower back, abdomen, legs and feet will help to strengthen the Ki in the legs. Such a person would also benefit from regular exercise with the legs, such as walking, jogging, cycling, or sports using the legs like football. This will draw Ki into the Hara and legs and strengthen them. Eating a lot of Yin foods has often contributed to this weakness, so a balanced diet with little or no sugar, spices, tea, coffee or tropical fruits will allow this area to become stronger.

The thighs reflect the strength of a person's sexual energy, especially the inside of the thigh. If this area is weak a person may develop knock knees. Extra Shiatsu here will strengthen the legs and reproductive organs. Exercise using the legs and a balanced diet will help to strengthen the thighs, as described above.

The knees are particularly affected by the condition of the middle organs of the body, the liver, gall bladder, stomach (pancreas), spleen and kidneys. If there are pains, weakness or stiffness in the knees there is almost certainly an imbalance in these organs, which will also be reflected in the middle of the back and upper half of the abdomen. Pain in the front of the knees around the knee caps relates to the Stomach, Spleen and pancreas. Pain on the inside and outside of the knees relates more to the Liver and Gall Bladder, and pain at the back of the knee relates to the Kidneys.

Pain in the knees can be helped by using Kyo and Jitsu. If the area of pain feels weak, soft and empty, it needs to be tonified by holding the sensitive points. If the area is tense and full, it needs to be relaxed by moving the Energy away from the area. If you are not sure which to do, give a moderate amount of Shiatsu on the painful area, and above and below on the thigh and lower leg. There is a variety of dietary causes of knee pains, which are too detailed to explain here. A balanced diet will help most cases and can be recommended.

The calves reflect the health of the intestines, bladder and kidneys. If the calf muscles are painful when touched, or swollen or hard, it indicates that the intestines are not in a good condition. Shiatsu on the calves will help to get the Energy flowing in the intestines, and relax the calves as well. Reducing the more extreme Yin and Yang foods and eating more of the Energetically balanced foods will improve the health of the intestines and so improve the condition of the calves.

If a person frequently gets cramps in the calves and/or in the soles of the feet, there is an imbalance in the Kidney and Bladder Meridians. Shiatsu down the back and backs of the legs and on the soles of the feet often helps to remedy this problem. Cutting down on more extreme foods that have a detrimental effect on the health of the kidneys, especially excess salt and drinks like tea, coffee, alcohol and tropical fruit juices, will also improve kidney functioning and therefore help reduce the cramping.

The ankles are related to the kidneys and reproductive organs. Puffiness or swelling around the ankles is generally caused by the kidneys functioning poorly, so that excess fluid is not efficiently removed from the body. Shiatsu down the whole of the back of the body and around the ankles and on the soles of the feet can help, along with the dietary changes already mentioned above.

A person with weak ankles may be prone to twisting them and they may feel very sensitive when you give Shiatsu here. However, more Shiatsu is needed to strengthen the Energy in the ankles, though not enough to cause too much pain.

The Feet

The feet can tell us an amazing amount through Oriental diagnosis. The health of all the major organs in the body is reflected in the feet. The shape of the feet also particularly reflects the quality of our contact with the ground and with the practical realities in our life.

We use our feet to step forward in life. If the feet appear strong with a well-curved arch, a person's intestines and kidneys are probably functioning well, and they probably have a strong will and self-determination. They are likely to do a lot in life. If the feet appear rather lifeless, maybe with a weak arch making the foot look flat, there may be weakness in the kidneys and intestines and the person will tend to lack a firm footing in their life. An excess of more Yin foods is often one cause of this weakness. Firm Shiatsu to the ankles, soles and toes will help to Energize the feet and the whole body.

Sometimes the toes appear to be clasping the ground, and there is a lot of tension in the upper side of the feet. Usually the Liver and Gall Bladder Meridians, that run from the first and fourth toes up the top of the foot, are Jitsu, causing tension that pulls the toes into their clasping position. Generally, the liver and gall bladder have become too Yang from the consumption of a lot of meat, eggs, poultry and salt, so a reduction in these foods and a more balanced diet will improve the health of these organs and help the feet straighten. Shiatsu with the thumb along the grooves between the metatarsal bones on the upper side of the feet will help shift the excess Ki that has built up here, helping the toes straighten and enhancing the functioning of the liver and gall bladder. When the toes curl in this way, a person frequently has a rather rigid outlook on life, and resists changes. They may be happier if they can try to become more flexible and open-minded, and accept change and new ideas in their lives.

When some people lie on their back, their feet droop towards the floor, due to the upper side of the feet being Kyo. This indicates that the chest, Lungs and Heart are also Kyo. The person's spirit or sense of themselves may be low. Shiatsu to the feet and chest will be beneficial. Usually they have consumed a lot of Yin foods and often lack regular physical exercise. A balanced diet with little of the extreme Yin foods will help to strengthen the chest. Encouragement to express inner feelings and desires may also be appropriate.

The Abdomen

Like the back, the abdomen reflects the health of the whole person. The quality of Energy in the twelve Meridians can be diagnosed in the abdomen by a skilled Shiatsu practitioner. At this stage in learning Shiatsu, we are going to look more generally at the abdomen and what you can easily diagnose now.

The lower half of the abdomen from the navel downwards reflects the strength of the Hara, the centre of Energy and vitality for the whole body and being. The Energetic condition is generally the same as the area directly behind it, the lower back, so if during your Shiatsu you found the lower back to be weak, then the Hara will probably also be weak.

Ideally, this centre should be full of Ki, which creates a slight bulge in the lower abdomen (not the whole abdomen!) with a bouncy, resilient but not hard or tense feel to the area. Such a person will probably have a lot of physical and mental energy, a healthy sexual drive, and a strong centredness and confidence. If the lower abdomen is weak, you will find that you can push into it easily with little resistance. The person may be feeling fatigued or stressed. Pushing in and holding in the lower abdomen will help draw Ki into the Hara, and also strengthen the kidneys and intestines. A weak Hara is often created by eating a lot of Yin foods like sugar, fruits, tea and coffee. A balanced diet with plenty of whole grains, vegetables, sea vegetables and soups seasoned with miso will help to strengthen the Hara. Physical exercise using the legs can also be helpful.

When you are giving Shiatsu to the centre of the abdomen around the navel, pushing in deeply with your fingers, you will feel the small intestine. Often on pushing in, your fingers will hit what feels like a rock inside. This is tension in the intestine, which is mostly muscle, and like any muscle on the outside of the body, it can become chronically tense and hard. Obviously when the intestine is cramped like this, digestion cannot be so efficient, and the Energy being held here would be more useful circulating around the whole body. Tension in the intestines can be caused by withholding emotions, and also by a poor diet. Gentle holding on this tense area will often result in it relaxing, releasing a lot of Energy and inner tension.

The upper half of the abdomen above the navel contains the middle organs, the liver, gall bladder, stomach, spleen and pancreas. This area should be flexible, so that your fingers can sink in deeply under the ribs. Unfortunately this is often not the case; the area is more often hard due to a build-up and stagnation of Energy. A typical modern diet containing animal products, sugar and refined foods creates a stagnation of Energy in these organs. This area also reflects the solar plexus Chakra, the centre of personal power. Repressing one's feelings and emotions over a long period of time creates a build-up of tension in this area and in the diaphragm, the sheet of muscle that separates the chest cavity from the abdominal cavity. Shiatsu to the upper abdomen and over the lower ribs when giving Shiatsu to the chest helps release this tension. You may have to be patient in slowly getting the accumulated Ki to move out of the area.

Some people find it almost unbearable to have their abdomen touched by another person. They might feel threatened and vulnerable even by the thought of being touched here. These people generally have a great deal of unresolved emotional tension held in the abdomen, and their fear is actually of releasing these emotions so that they have to experience and face up to them. It is obviously desirable that they should do this, but great sensitivity and compassion will be needed. Be prepared for them bursting into tears!

The Chest

The chest reflects the health of the heart and the circulation, and also the heart Chakra which is the centre of love, compassion and feeling. In Chinese teachings, the Heart is the store place of Shen, our individual spirit that guides us through life. When it is active we feel happy and alive; when it is relatively inactive we feel sad and dead. The Heart of small children is usually 'open', and they feel a lot and are alive and spirited, as well as being vulnerable. During our life we frequently 'close' our Heart to protect it against being hurt. But as it closes, so does our ability to feel, to live, and be alive.

Often the chest looks collapsed or hollow, and the person may look resigned and in need of support. Their circulation is generally weak, giving a pale complexion. The chest then needs to be treated sensitively; rough Shiatsu could cause the Heart to close further. Gentle but firm Shiatsu, with more holding to bring Ki into this area, can help the chest and Heart open. The person may like to share some of the feelings that have caused their Hearts to close. Exercise involving deep breathing can also help by bringing more Ki into the chest.

Sometimes the chest appears over-inflated, expanded and Jitsu. The circulation is often over-active, possibly resulting in high blood pressure. Such a person can seem confident and assertive, but underneath they may be frightened of letting go. Shiatsu can help move the excess Energy out of the area, and loosen the muscles so that the chest relaxes.

The Arms

As a whole the arms and hands are mainly fed by Energy from the heart and throat Chakras, so the strength of Ki in the arms is closely connected with what is happening in the chest. For example, when the chest is Kyo, the arms and hands are usually weak also. The arms and hands could be called 'the wings of the Heart'; they are used for giving and receiving, and also in expressing our feelings. When giving Shiatsu to the arms it can be useful to consider them along with the chest – if the chest, arms and hands are Kyo as a whole then they all need to be tonified; if they are all Jitsu then they all need to be sedated.

The inside of the upper arm is especially connected with the heart as the Heart Meridian passes along here. (Interestingly, this is where pain is usually first felt during a heart attack.) If this area seems particularly weak and flabby, the Heart Meridian is low in Energy, and extra Shiatsu to this area will be beneficial.

The elbows, like the knees, are associated with the middle organs of the body: the liver, gall bladder, stomach, spleen and pancreas. Pains or other problems around the elbows are usually associated with an Energy imbalance in the middle organs, which can also be diagnosed in the middle back, upper abdomen, knees and feet. If there are pains in the elbows, such as in tennis elbow, you can give Shiatsu to the painful places, if possible diagnosing whether they are Kyo or Jitsu and treating them appropriately. The dietary causes of the pain are various, so apart from eating the balanced diet, recommendations cannot be given here.

The wrists, like the ankles, are Energetically connected with the kidneys and reproductive organs. A person's wrists may look weak, making them prone to spraining or breaking them. The skin may also be darker around the wrist than on the rest of the arm, especially on the inside of the arm. This indicates poor health in the kidneys and reproductive organs. When the wrists are weak, extra time can be spent giving Shiatsu to them, especially pressing with the thumb into the groove between the bones of the lower arm and those of the hand.

The Hands

The hands as a whole are closely connected to the heart and circulation, although like the feet they also reflect the health condition of all the organs of the body. If the hands overall appear weak and rather lifeless, the person's Heart Energy and circulation are probably also weak. They may have difficulties with their emotional expression, with giving and receiving. Firm Shiatsu to the palms and fingers can help Energize the hands, warm the heart and improve circulation.

On the other hand the hands may be very warm, possibly red, swollen and tense. The Heart and circulation are probably over-active, and the person tense overall. With an over-active Heart there may also be a tendency to high blood pressure. Shiatsu over the hands and fingers can draw some of this excess Energy off, relieving the tension and helping the person feel calmer and more relaxed.

This chapter has given you a lot of information which hopefully will provide a basis for your continued experimentation with giving Shiatsu. As you progress to perceiving and working with imbalances in different areas of the body, don't lose sight of the overall needs of a person. There is a danger of becoming preoccupied with giving Shiatsu to detailed areas and losing touch with the needs of an individual as a whole. You may then be effective in working on particular areas, but the overall effect may not be so good. So try to keep in mind the wider needs of your friend while you are giving Shiatsu.

CHAPTER 11

Incorporating Tsubos into your Shiatsu

In this chapter, a number of the Tsubos or acupuncture points most commonly used in acupuncture, acupressure and Shiatsu are listed, with their numbers, names in English, and precise location and common uses. Particular points have specific effects due to a number of Energetic relationships with the rest of the body.

1 A Tsubo frequently has an effect on the Energy in its surrounding area. For example, a number of points around the shoulder are useful for relieving pain and other problems in the shoulder.

2 Giving Shiatsu to a Tsubo affects the Energy flow along the Meridian that it lies on. A Tsubo may thus be useful for a problem that is associated with an imbalance of Energy in another part of its Meridian. For example, Large Intestine 4 in the hand can be used to help alleviate toothache as this Meridian runs from the hand to the face.

3 Tsubos can be used to create changes in the internal Organs of the body, via the Meridian they lie on. So Lung 1 on the inside of the shoulder can benefit lung problems like asthma and coughing, and Large Intestine 4 can help constipation and other large intestine problems.

4 There are a number of other relationships between specific Tsubos and the rest of the body, based on more complex Oriental theories than this introductory book can cover. Some of the books given in the Further Reading section can be consulted for this information.

You can use the following list in two ways. Firstly, if you yourself or somebody you are going to treat has a particular health problem, consult the list and find any points that are indicated as being commonly useful for that problem. Look at the location of the Tsubo on the charts and read the description of their location, and then find them either on your own or on the receiver's body. From the chart and description you should be able to get quite close to the actual Tsubo on the body, but to find it precisely you now need to 'feel about' until you sense you are right on it. Very often when you precisely locate a Tsubo, your thumb or finger 'falls' into a little depression, and the point feels more sensitive than the surrounding area when pressed. You may also just intuitively feel, 'I've got it!'

For another person, these Tsubos are ideally incorporated into their full-body Shiatsu treatment. Give Shiatsu to the Tsubos as you come to them in your full-body treatment, rather than working on them separately. If you do not have the time to give a full treatment, you could just apply pressure to the points, but the receiver will get much more benefit if you also give them a full-body treatment. If you are using Tsubos on yourself, you will unfortunately only be able to use the points!

The second way of using this list is that while giving Shiatsu, you will discover points that feel as if they particularly need holding. These points are often, but by no means always, recognized acupuncture points. You can consult the list to see if these points are recognized acupuncture points, and if so, check their names, numbers and common uses. In this way you can learn from the body of knowledge built up from other people's experience.

I would recommend using this list in both of these ways. Over-dependence on the first method can stunt the development of your own sensitivity and trust in what you discover through touching the body. As your sense of touch develops, you will actually find the points on a particular person's body that are most in need of Shiatsu, and that will give the greatest benefits. Trust what you feel through your touch more than what you read in a book!

When you use specific Tsubos, use the points on both sides of the body. The points can be held for anything from a half a minute to two minutes. Apply pressure while observing the Basic Principles for giving Shiatsu described in Chapter 5. In particular, make sure that your pressure is exactly at right-angles to the body surface at the point. Then your Ki penetrates to the bottom of the Tsubo and has the maximum beneficial effect. Even if the angle is only slightly out, you will not reach the bottom, and the effect is greatly reduced.

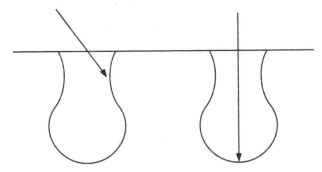

Fig. 77 Pressure at Right-angles Reaches the Bottom of Tsubos

When you press a Tsubo you may feel that the Energy at the point is full, with greater muscle tone, or more Jitsu. You then need to press the point in such a way as to disperse the excess Energy. Simple holding may be enough, or you may find that making small circular movements with your thumb or 'pumping' your thumb in and out is more effective, until you feel the excess Energy subside and the excess muscle tone relax. On the other hand, Energy at the point may be lacking, so that the Tsubo feels deficient, 'needy', and unusually soft. Energy needs to be brought into such Kyo points, by simply holding them for some time. As you hold you may well be able to feel the point 'filling up' with Energy, and the muscle tone increasing slightly. For more detailed information on the diagnosis and treatment of Kyo and Jitsu, refer back to Chapter 8.

There are some points that should not be used during pregnancy, as they give strong stimulation to the uterus and could cause a miscarriage. These are clearly marked in the list, so please avoid them if there is any possibility of your receiver being pregnant.

In describing the location of Tsubos the Oriental term 'cun' is used. 1 cun is the width of the receiver's thumb at the widest point. The width of the receiver's four fingers is approximately 3 cun. If your hands are about the same size as the receiver's, you can use your own fingers to make these measurements.

Fig. 78 Using the Fingers to Measure Cun

LG Lung
LI Large Intestine
ST Stomach
SP Spleen
HT Heart
SI Small Intestine
BL Bladder
KD Kidney
HG Heart Governor
TH Triple Heater
GB Gall Bladder
LV Liver
GV Governing Vessel
CV Conception Vessel

Front view

Back view

Front view

Back view

Fig. 79 Charts for Finding the Tsubo

t view

Back view

LG Lung
LI Large Intestine
ST Stomach
SP Spleen
HT Heart
SI Small Intestine
BL Bladder
KD Kidney
HG Heart Governor
TH Triple Heater
GB Gall Bladder
LV Liver
GV Governing Vessel
CV Conception Vessel

Number Name in English	Location	Common Uses
LUNG		
1 Centre of Gathering	Between 1st and 2nd ribs, 1 cun below middle of collar bone	Asthma, coughs, common cold, breathing difficulties, pain in chest, shoulder pain
5 In the Groove	On end of elbow crease on thumb side of arm	Elbow pain and swelling, tonsilitis, painful breathing, coughs, asthma, fever associated with lung problems
7 Broken Sequence	1½ cun above wrist crease on thumb side of arm	Congestion, headaches, colds, coughing, Bells palsy, stiff neck
9 Great Stagnation	On wrist crease in indentation below thumb	Reviving unconscious person, coughs, painful breathing, pharyngitis, pain and paralysis of wrist
LARGE INTESTINE		
4 Great Eliminator	On tip of fleshy mound which is formed by drawing thumb into index finger	Normalizes intestines, general wellbeing, facial problems, e.g. frontal headache, neuralgia, lower toothache, problems of back of hand **Don't use during pregnancy**
10 Arm Three Miles	1½ cun below the end of the crease formed by bending elbow	Sore throat, general well-being, pain or fatigue in arms
11 Lake of Energy on the Corner	End of crease formed by bending elbow	Hypertension, tennis elbow, haemorrhoids
15 Corner of the Shoulder	In indentation on outside of shoulder bone	Frozen shoulder, neuralgia of arm and shoulder, hemiplegia
20 Welcome Fragrance	In groove at wide point of nostrils	Sinusitis, facial tension, neuralgia of face, paralysis of facial nerves
STOMACH		
3 Empty Space in Bone	Directly below pupil in space under cheekbone	Sinus and nasal congestion, facial tension or paralysis, upper toothache, neuralgia of face

25 Heavenly Pivot	2 cun either side of the navel	Abdominal pain, menstrual pain, bowel irregularities, intestinal obstruction
36 Leg Three Miles	In depression outside the tibia 3 cun below the kneecap	Well-being, particularly for tonifying Stomach and Spleen Meridians, fatigue, tired legs, loss of appetite
44 Inner Garden	Between 2nd and 3rd toe division, pushing in towards 2nd toe	Stomach pain, toothache, frontal headache, sore throat

SPLEEN

6 Meeting Point of the Three Yin Leg Meridians	3 cun above the tip of ankle bone, push in to the edge of the tibia	Ankle pains, menstrual pain, digestive problems, female reproductive problems, insomnia, overweight **Don't use during pregnancy**
10 Ocean of Blood	3 cun above the kneecap on bulge of muscle	Itching, hives, menstrual pain

HEART

7 Gate of God	On wrist crease in indentation below little finger	Reviving unconscious person, insomnia, hysteria, high blood pressure, irritability, angina pectoris
9 Little Rushing In	Inside the little finger about 0.1 cun from the corner of the nail	Heart attack, severe anxiety, hysteria, angina pectoris

SMALL INTESTINE

3 Back Stream	On crease formed by making a fist on edge of hand below little finger	Paralysis of fingers, numbness, hardness of hearing, ringing in ears
11 Centre of Heaven	Two thirds up midline of shoulder blade	Shoulder pain, frozen shoulder, intercostal neuralgia, lung problems
19 Palace of Hearing	In the depression between the jaw joint and the middle part of the ear	Ringing in ears, difficulty in hearing

BLADDER

1 Eye Brightness	Inner corner of eye	Poor or tired vision, swollen eyes
2 Collecting Bamboo	In notch directly above Bladder 1	Front or back headache, hay fever, eye strain

10	Pillar of Heaven	Below back of skull, 1 cun to the sides of the middle of the neck	Headaches, insomnia, nasal congestion, neck ache, eye and nose problems
13	Lung Back Transporting Point	1.5 cun to the sides of the spine, level with the space between the 3rd and 4th thoracic vertebrae	Cough, asthma, breathlessness, bronchitis, pneumonia. Tonifies deficient Lungs
23	Kidney Back Transporting Point	1.5 cun to the sides of the spine level with the space between the 2nd and 3rd lumbar vertebrae	Tonifies Kidneys, impotence, infertility, lack of sexual desire, physical weakness and exhaustion, depression, lack of will-power, chronic low back pain, weak legs, chronic ear problems, e.g. tinnitus, deafness; poor vision
24	Sea of Ki Back Transporting Point	1.5 cun to the sides of the space between the 3rd and 4th lumbar vertebrae	Chronic or acute lower back pain, irregular menstruation, uterine bleeding
25	Large Intestine Back Transporting Point	1.5 cun to the sides of the space between the 4th and 5th lumbar vertebrae	Tonifies Large Intestine, constipation or diarrhoea, abdominal distension, chronic or acute lower back pain
27	Small Intestine Back Transporting Point	At level of 1st depression in the sacrum, 1.5 cun out from the centre of the sacrum	Any small intestine problem, e.g. abdominal pain; back pain over sacrum, urination and menstruation problems
28	Bladder Back Transporting Point	At level of 2nd depression in the sacrum, 1.5 cun out from the centre of the sacrum	Bladder problems, e.g. difficult urination, retention of urine, bed-wetting; strengthens lower back
40	Supporting Middle	In middle of crease behind knee	Lower backache, calf spasms, sciatica
57	In the Mountain	In depression in centre of calf muscle	Sciatica, tired legs, calf spasms, pain on sole of foot
60	Mountain	On the outside of the ankle between the ankle bone and Achilles tendon	Sciatica, dizziness, backache **Don't use during pregnancy**
67	Extreme Yin	Outside of the little toe, at base of toenail	Malposition of foetus, headaches, blurred vision, pain in eyes and other eye problems **Don't use during pregnancy**

KIDNEY

1 Bubbling Spring	In the crease in the middle of the ball of the foot	General vitality, fear, dizziness, revival
3 Greater Stream	Between tip of ankle bone and Achilles tendon	General kidney function, pain in lower back, impotence, abnormal menstruation, deficient Kidney Energy
27 Transportation Place	Between 1st rib and collar bone	Bronchitis, chest pain, asthma

HEART GOVERNOR

6 Inside Gate	2 cun above wrist crease between tendons in the middle of the forearm	Nausea, vomiting, sea sickness, insomnia, heart palpitations
8 Palace of Anxiety	Cup hand; at bottom of the 'cup' in the palm	Exhaustion, shyness, high blood pressure, writer's cramp

TRIPLE HEATER

5 Outer Gate	2 cun above wrist crease on back of arm	Tinnitus, ear infection, migraine headaches, aversion to cold
14 Top of Shoulder	Just behind the tip of the shoulder bone	Shoulder joint pain
23 Silk Bamboo Hollow	At outside tip of eyebrow in depression on bone around eye	Headache, eye and ear problems

GALL BLADDER

1 Hole in Bone for Eye	Outside corner of eye in depression on bone around eye	Headache around temples, conjunctivitis, eye problems
12 Whole Bone	Depression below the back edge of the skull and behind the bone behind the ear	Headache, toothache, ringing in ear
14 Pure Yang	1 cun above the middle of the eyebrow	Front headaches, sinus blockage, eye problems
20 Windy Pond	Below the back edge of the skull, between the back and side neck muscles	Eye disorders, common cold, front and side headaches, hypertension, tension in neck, dizziness, vertigo

21 Shoulder Well	A little behind the highest point of the shoulder in line with the 7th cervical vertebra	Shoulder pain, frozen shoulder, mastitis, lack of milk, childbirth difficulties **Don't use during pregnancy**
30 Jumping Circle	One-third of the way between the head of the femur and the coccyx in the side of the buttocks	Sciatica, lumbar pain, lumbago, arthritis or rheumatism in hip area, hip problems
34 Yang Hill Spring	In the depression behind and below the head of the fibula	Ankle pains, headaches, knee problems, leg weakness
40 Mound Ruins	In depression in front of and slightly below the ankle bone	Lumbago, aids function of liver and gall bladder, neck pain, calf pain

LIVER

3 Bigger Rushing	1½ cun above bridge of 1st and 2nd toes	Headaches, dizziness, muscle cramps and muscle tension
8 Spring on the Corner	On inside of knee joint, above bent knee crease	Inside knee problems, urine retention, burning urination, itchy genitals
14 Gate of Hope	Between 6th and 7th ribs directly below nipple	Rib pain, lactation problems, coughing, breathing difficulty

GOVERNING VESSEL

4 Gate of Life	Between 2nd and 3rd lumbar vertebrae	Strengthens Kidneys, lumbar weakness, lack of vitality, impotence, infertility, weak legs
12 Body Pillar	Between 3rd and 4th thoracic vertebrae	Asthma, colds, calms nervous system, strengthens whole body
14 Big Vertebra	Between 7th cervical and 1st thoracic vertebrae	Common cold, fever, asthma, headaches, clears mind and stimulates brain
15 Gate of Fool	Between 1st and 2nd cervical vertebrae	Colds, headaches, nosebleeds; stimulates speech, so good for speech difficulties
16 Wind Palace	Between skull and 1st cervical vertebra	Stimulates/calms brain, giddiness, tension in upper neck

20 Hundred Meetings	At the centre of head on middle of line connecting tops of ears	Headaches, giddiness, piles, prolapsed anus or vagina

CONCEPTION VESSEL

4 Gate to Original Ki	3 cun below navel	Strengthens overall Ki and body and mind, deficient Kidney Energy, fatigue, grounding, reproductive organ problems
6 Ocean of Ki	1½ cun below navel	Physical and mental exhaustion and depression, lower abdominal pain or distension, lack of willpower
14 Great Palace	1 cun below lower tip of breastbone	Acts on stomach and heart, stomach spasm, stomach ulcers, emotional upset, calms mind
17 Middle of Chest	On breastbone directly between nipples	Acts on heart and lungs. Pain or fullness in chest, breathlessness, chronic cough or bronchitis, palpitations, high blood pressure, asthma, angina pectoris
22 Heaven Projection	Between the inside ends of the collar bones	Acute and chronic cough and asthma, bronchitis, sore throat

EXTRA POINTS NOT LYING ON MERIDIANS

Yintang Seal Hall	Between the eyebrows	Calms mind and tension in forehead, frontal headaches, blocked frontal sinuses
Taiyang Greater Yang	In depression 1 cun behind the middle of the outer end of the eyebrow and outer corner of the eye	Headaches in the side of the head, over-active mind, eye problems
Xiyan Knee Eyes	Two points in the depressions at the lower outside corners of the kneecap	Pain in front of knee or deep inside joint

CHAPTER 12

Meridian Exercises for Yourself

This chapter describes some stretching exercises, called Makko-ho exercises, that promote Energy flow in the twelve main Meridians. They are widely taught along with Shiatsu as a way of improving health, and of assessing the condition of the Energy flow within one's own Meridians. They are quite simple and take about ten minutes to run through. Ideally they can be practised daily, for example in the morning after getting up. They can also be used as a part of other exercise programmes, or at any time of the day when the body feels in need of some rejuvenation.

There are six exercises, each stretching one pair of Meridians. Stretching a Meridian has the effect of stimulating Energy to flow along that Meridian. By stretching all the Meridians with the six exercises, one's entire Energy flow through the Meridian system is improved. This often has the benefits of removing tiredness (which is often due to stuck Energy flow rather than a lack of Energy as often thought) and making the body feel lighter. Stretching the Meridians also has the effect of rebalancing the Energy flow in the Meridian system: if a Meridian is Jitsu, the stretch helps to move the excess Energy out; if it is Kyo, more Energy will be brought in.

In order to promote Energy flow, these exercises must be done in a particular way. Many other stretching exercises are performed for a physical effect, and it is thought best to stretch as far as possible regardless of the tension and pain this may produce. The body may also be 'bounced' to stretch that little bit further. While this kind of stretching may increase physical flexibility, it has little effect on Energy flow, as pain and tension prevent the flow of Energy. (You will find that practising the Makko-ho exercises is actually a very effective way of increasing your flexibility, painlessly.)

The Makko-ho exercises are performed quite differently so as to have the maximum effect on Energy. Firstly you stay relaxed throughout, with smooth, continuous breathing. You only move into the stretch position as far as is needed to feel a stretch in the particular Meridian pair, without any force, so that you can stay relaxed. Secondly, the stretch is held for some time, from half a minute to several minutes, to give time for the Energy to move, rather than a quick 'in and out' motion. After holding a particular stretch for 5, 10 or 15 seconds, you may feel any stiffness or slight pain beginning to recede, and the stretch becomes much easier. This is the moment when Ki begins to flow. Once Energy starts flowing you obviously want to hold the stretch longer so that as much Energy as possible is set moving. With a quick stretch or bouncing movement, this moment is never reached.

Besides the health benefits of the Makko-ho exercises, they can also be used to assess the relative condition of your six pairs of Meridians. If you feel a lot of stiffness and resistance with a restricted amount of movement in a particular stretch, it indicates that the pair of Meridians is more Jitsu. On the other hand if a stretch is easier with a greater amount of movement, and feels particularly pleasurable, the Meridian pair being stretched is probably more Kyo. Some people who generally find stretching exercises very easy actually have a lot of Kyo Meridians. When you run through all six stretches, it will probably become clear which of your Meridian pairs are most out of balance. If you practise the Makko-ho exercises regularly you will be able to observe these most imbalanced Meridians gradually coming into balance. You may also like to practise the stretches for your most imbalanced Meridians more often, to produce a quicker rebalancing and improvement in your health.

The Makko-ho exercises can also be used as a basis for other stretching-type exercises. Once you are familiar with the location of the Meridians, you can experiment with yoga asanas and other exercises to see which Meridians they most effectively stretch. You can then select other stretching exercises to work on particular Meridians.

How to Perform the Exercises

1 Before you begin the exercises, make sure that you are relaxed and centred. You could practise abdominal breathing (see Chapter 5) for a few minutes before you begin.

2 Before each stretch, take a breath in, then breathe out as you go into the stretch. As you hold the stretch position, keep breathing evenly and continuously. Holding the breath holds tension in the body, whereas with continuous breathing tension is released on each out breath. Then as you rise out of the stretch, take a deep breath in, then breathe out and relax.

3 Only move as far into each stretch position as you can without creating discomfort and tension throughout your body. You should be able to feel a stretch along the pair of Meridians, but this should not be so much as to cause pain.

4 Hold the stretch for half a minute to several minutes. See if you can feel the moment at which Energy begins to move, and the position begins to feel more comfortable. As more Energy flows you may well find that you can move a little further into the stretch.

5 After completing all six exercises, a lot of Energy will have been set moving. If you immediately jump up and start rushing about, you will stop this movement, so it is a good idea to lie down for a few minutes to allow the Energy to keep flowing and come to a new balance. When you feel ready, get up and try to keep the feeling of being relaxed and centred as you go about your day's activities.

Lung and Large Intestine Meridian Stretch

Stand with your feet shoulder width apart, hook your thumbs together behind your back and stretch your fingers outwards. As you breathe out, bend forwards, keeping the legs and arms straight. Bring your hands as far over the head as possible without using force – imagine that somebody else is pulling your hands forward. The feeling should be of an enjoyable stretch. Check your body to make sure that you are not tensing up, and breathe slowly as you hold the position for half a minute or more. You may well be able to feel a particularly strong stretch along the Lung and Large Intestine Meridians in the shoulders, arms and thumbs. Finally breathe in as you slowly straighten up to a standing position.

Fig. 80

Spleen and Stomach Meridian Stretch

Kneel on the floor, and move your feet outwards so that your bottom sits on the floor. If your bottom does not reach the floor, put a cushion under it so that your body weight is resting through your bottom on the floor. Now, as you breathe out, lean backwards and support your weight on your hands behind you. You may now feel a stretch along the Spleen and Stomach Meridians on the front of your thighs and lower legs. If it feels that you are getting plenty of stretch in this position and that you could not comfortably stretch any further, stay in this position for at least half a minute, breathing evenly.

If you feel that you need to stretch further, drop down onto your elbows. Make sure your knees are within a few inches of each other and on the floor – if they splay outwards or upwards the Meridians are not so effectively stretched. Again, if this is as far as you can comfortably go, stay in this position; don't think that you have to force yourself further. It is so important to be able to stay relaxed while stretching. If, however, you feel that you could quite easily stretch further, drop your back onto the floor. Raise your arms over your head and interlock the fingers to increase the stretching of these Meridians in the abdomen and chest. If you feel discomfort or pain in your lower back, don't force yourself to stay in this position; go back to resting on your elbows. Otherwise, after half a minute or so, raise yourself back onto your elbows, then onto your hands, then sit up straight.

Heart and Small Intestine Meridian Stretch

Sit on the floor and draw the soles of your feet together. Grasp your feet with your hands and pull the feet as close to the body as possible. Make sure your elbows are outside your legs, and as you breathe out lean forward, taking your head towards or onto your feet. Hold this position for at least half a minute, breathing evenly. This is not such a strenuous stretch as the last two, but you will probably be able to feel a line of tension along the Heart and Small Intestine Meridians on the under-side of the arms. Finally breathe in as you rise out of the stretch position, and relax.

Kidney and Bladder Meridian Stretch

Sit on the floor with your legs straight out in front of you and bend forwards from the hips, reaching with your hands as far down the legs as you can comfortably go. You may be able to hold onto your feet or, if you cannot stretch that far, your ankles. Drop your head forwards to stretch the Bladder Meridian in the back of the neck. You should now be able to feel a line of stretch in the Kidney and Bladder Meridians all the way from your feet, up the backs of the legs, to the back and neck. Hold the position for half a minute or more as usual, making sure that your breathing is free and easy and your body is relaxed. Then rise back up to a sitting position as you breathe in.

Heart Governor and Triple Heater Meridian Stretch

Sit on the floor either with the soles of your feet together or with the feet crossed over each other, whichever is more comfortable. Now cross your arms over each other and grasp your knees with your hands wrapped well around the knees. Take a breath in, and then as you breathe out drop your head and body forwards and your knees downwards towards the floor so that the hands are pulled away from each other. You should now feel a stretch along the front and back of the arms along the pathways of the Heart Governor and Triple Heater Meridians. Hold for half a minute or so, breathing evenly, then breathe in and rise back up to a sitting position.

Liver and Gall Bladder Meridian Stretch

Sitting on the floor, spread your legs as wide apart as they will comfortably go, while keeping them straight. Bending from the waist, reach down one leg with your hand as far as is comfortable, and bring the other arm over your head towards the same foot. Keep facing forwards rather than facing the leg, so that the side of your torso is stretched. Relax and breathe evenly. You should now be able to feel the pathways of the Liver and Gall Bladder Meridians being stretched on the inside and outside of the legs and in the side of the torso.

After holding for half a minute or more, breathe in as you sit up again, then breathe out and go down to the other leg. Again hold for at least half a minute while breathing evenly, then rise back up to a sitting position.

Now that you have finished the six exercises, lie down on your back with your arms to your sides for a few minutes. Relax and tune into what is happening within your body. You may well be able to feel sensations of Energy moving around your body. When you feel ready, you can get up.

Postscript

I hope that you have enjoyed this book, that the information has brought a new way of looking at your life and health, and that you have now given lots of Shiatsu to your friends. There is a lot of information in Part 3 that will take time for you to appreciate fully and put into practice, so you may well like to go back over this part of the book.

If you have enjoyed learning Shiatsu I encourage you to learn more by attending some classes with a qualified teacher. It is a great help in learning this very practical art to be taught at first hand. The Useful Addresses section at the end of this book has a list of the major schools running Shiatsu courses in Britain. If none of these are close to you, try contacting the Shiatsu Society which has a longer list of teachers. There are also a number of teachers and centres where you can find out more about food Energetics and its therapeutic uses. The Community Health Foundation can supply a list of contacts throughout the country.

Glossary

Anma A traditional form of massage used in Japan.

Astral body The subtle Energetic body associated with our emotions.

Aura The extension of the body's Energy beyond the physical body. Consists of a number of 'layers': the etheric, astral, mental and causal.

Barley malt A sweetener made from sprouted barley grains. Also called malt extract, it is used to sweeten cakes, biscuits and other desserts, porridge, drinks, etc.

Causal body The subtle Energetic body associated with a person's soul or 'higher self'.

Chakra A wheel or centre of Energy within the Energetic body. There are seven main Chakras lying on the spiritual channel, and many more minor Chakras.

Energy Subtle Energy detectable by living organisms but not by mechanical instruments, to be distinguished from the Western idea of energy which is associated with matter. Called Ki in Japanese.

Etheric body The densest subtle body closely associated with the physical functioning of the body.

Fu An Organ concerned with transforming food and drink into Energy for the body to use, and with excretion. Usually associated with a hollow organ, e.g. the stomach.

Hara The Energetic centre in the lower abdomen.

Ki Ki is universal, found everywhere and in all things. It manifests in different ways to create physical forms and living organisms. In the human body it creates our physical, emotional, mental and spiritual being.

Kyo A deficiency in Energy.

Jitsu An excess of Energy.

Macrobiotics A reinterpretation of ancient Oriental philosophy and medicine, begun this century by George Ohsawa and now taught by Michio Kushi and other teachers. Emphasizes living in harmony with nature and universal laws, especially through eating an Energetically balanced diet.

Mental body The subtle Energetic body associated with the intellect, containing thoughtforms.

Meridian A channel of Energy travelling over the body's surface and internally through the organs of the body.

Miso A rich-tasting soya bean paste used for seasoning soups, stews and other vegetable dishes. Made by fermenting soya beans with grain and sea salt for over a year.

Moxibustion The application of heat to acupuncture points; for example, by burning a small amount of dried mugwort on the skin.

Organ A group of functions including that of a physical organ, but also of other bodily functions, an emotion, tissue, sense organ and aspect of consciousness.

Spiritual channel A channel of Energy running between the top of the head and the base of the torso. The seven main Chakras lie on the spiritual channel.

Subtle body An Energetic body overlying the physical body and extending beyond the physical body to form the aura.

Tsubo A point on the skin where the Energy flow of a Meridian or of the body can be beneficially affected. 'Tsubo' is used to denote (a) an acupuncture point, and (b) any point on the body where Energy flow can be beneficially changed.

Yang Any phenomenon or form in which Energy is primarily contracting or becoming more organized, e.g. animals, growth, work, introversion.

Yin Any phenomenon or form in which Energy is primarily expanding or becoming more dispersed, e.g. decay, relaxation, expression.

Zang An Organ concerned with the storage of Energy, and usually associated with a solid organ, e.g. the liver.

Further Reading

The Human Energetic Constitution
The Book of Do-in: Exercises for Physical and Spiritual Development, Michio Kushi. Japan Publications Inc., 1979.
Vibrational Medicine, Richard Gerber. Bear & Company, 1988.
The Yellow Emperor's Classic of Internal Medicine, Ilza Veith. University of California Press, 1966.

Shiatsu
Do-It-Yourself Shiatsu, Wataru Ohashi. Allen & Unwin, 1977.
The Book of Shiatsu, Saul Goodman. Avery, 1991.
Zen Shiatsu, Shizuto Masunaga and Wataru Ohashi, Japan Publications Inc., 1977.
Shiatsu: The Complete Guide, Chris Jarmey and Gabriel Mojay. Thorsons, 1991.

Food Energetics
An Introduction To Macrobiotics, Oliver Cowmeadow. Thorsons, 1987.
Yin Yang Cookbook, Oliver and Michele Cowmeadow. Macdonald Optima, 1988.
Food For Thought: A New Look at Food and Behaviour, Saul Miller with Jo Anne Miller. Prentice-Hall Inc., 1985.
Food and Healing, Annemarie Colbin. Ballantine Books, 1986.

Oriental Diagnosis
Your Face Never Lies: An Introduction to Oriental Diagnosis, Michio Kushi. Avery Publishing Group Inc., 1983.
How To See Your Health: Book of Oriental Diagnosis, Michio Kushi. Japan Publications Inc., 1980.
Your Body Speaks Its Mind, Stanley Keleman. The Centre Press, 1981.
Macrobiotics and Human Behaviour, William Tara. Japan Publications Inc., 1984.

Useful Addresses

If you would like to study Shiatsu further, the following schools run introductory and longer professional training courses.

The Bristol School of Shiatsu and Oriental Medicine
81 Cornwall Road
Bishopston, Bristol
BS7 8LJ
01272 425680/772809

The British School Of Shiatsu-Do
East West Centre
188 Old Street
London EC1V 9BP
0171 251 0831

The Devon School of Shiatsu
The Coach House
Buckyette Farm
Littlehempston, Totnes
Devon TQ9 6ND
0180426 593

The East Anglia School of Shiatsu
2 Capondale Cottages
New Lane, Holbrook
Ipswich, Suffolk IP9 2RB
01473 328061

The European School of Shiatsu
High Banks, Lockeridge
Marlborough
Wiltshire SN8 4EQ
01672 86459

Glasgow School of Shiatsu
19 Langside Park
Kilbarchan
Renfrewshire PA10 2EP
015057 4657

Healing-Shiatsu Education Centre
The Orchard
Lower Maescoed
Hereford HR2 0HP
0187387 207

Ki Kai Shiatsu Centre
8 Willow Road,
Hampstead
London NW3
0181 368 9050

The London College of Massage and Shiatsu
6 Claribel Road
London SW9 6TH
0171 978 8150

The Natural Living and Healing Centre
Lios Dana, Inch,
Co. Kerry, Ireland
010 353 6658189

The Shiatsu College
20a Lower Goat Lane
Norwich, Norfolk
NR2 1EL
01603 632555

The American Shiatsu Society
44 Pearl Street
Cambridge MA 02139
USA

For further information on Shiatsu, or to find a Shiatsu therapist in your area, contact:

The Shiatsu Society
The Interchange Studios
Dalby Street
London NW5 3NQ
Tel: 0171 813 7772
Fax: 0171 813 7773

For information on classes in food Energetics and macrobiotics and therapists who give dietary consultations, contact:

The Community Health Foundation
188 Old Street
London EC1V 9BP
0171 251 4076

Index

abdomen
  in diagnosis 113, 115,
    119, 122–3
  problems 134, 135, 138
  technique 40, 70–1
abdominal centre *see*
  Hara
aches and pains 42
acupuncture 6, 7, 8, 23,
  27, 126, 127
Ajna *see* Brow Chakra
angina pectoris 134, 138
ankles
  in diagnosis 114, 120,
    121
  problems 134, 137
  technique 40, 65
Anma 7
anxiety 9, 110, 134
arms
  in diagnosis 111, 115,
    124–5
  problems 133
  technique 74–6, 130
arthritis 137
asthma 115, 126, 133, 135,
  136, 137, 138
astral body 15, 16, 109
aura 14–15, 32
autonomic nervous system
  23, 98

back
  in diagnosis 114–18
  problems 26, 42, 110,
    116, 117–18, 135, 136,
    137
  technique 52, 55, 60–1
Base Chakra 19, 20, 111,
  112, 119
Bells palsy 133

Bladder 22
  in diagnosis 110, 111,
    112, 118, 120
  Meridian 25, 26, 120,
    144
  problems 135, 137
  Tsubos 130–2, 134–5
body
  back/front 110–13
  bottom/top 113–14
  Tsubos 131
body reading 108–25
bowels, problems 134
breathing
  abdominal 45–9, 141
  problems 115, 116–17,
    124, 133, 135, 137,
    138
  recipient 59
bronchitis 115, 135, 136,
  138
Brow Chakra 19, 20, 46
buttocks 63, 113, 118

calves 120, 135, 137
causal body 16, 109
centred movement 50–6
Chakras 19–21
chest
  in diagnosis 113, 115,
    117, 121, 122, 123
  problems 133, 136, 138
  technique 72–3
Chi *see* Ki
childbirth 40, 135, 137
children 54, 87
circulation
  in diagnosis 111, 112,
    115, 116–17, 123, 124,
    125
  problems 134, 136, 138
  colds 42, 133, 136, 137

Conception Vessel 23, 24,
  130–2, 138
conjunctivitis 136
constipation 115, 126, 135
coughing 42, 126, 133,
  135, 137, 138
Crown Chakra 19, 20
cun 129

diagnosis 89–90, 108–25
diarrhoea 115, 135
diet
  balanced 105–7, 108
  beneficial changes
    108–25
  Energetic qualities
    93–102, 105–7, 108
  fat deposits 44
  traditional 102–5
  Yin and Yang 96–102
digestive system 40, 110,
  113, 134
Directing Vessel *see*
  Conception Vessel
dizziness 135, 136, 137

ears 134, 135, 136
elbows 124, 133
elderly people 43, 54, 87
emotions 26
  astral body 15, 16
  problems 26, 41, 110,
    115–16, 117, 123, 135,
    138
  release 43
Energy
  see also Ki
  blocked 28, 29, 139
  centres 45–6
  flow 8, 23, 26, 27–8, 52,
    89, 126, 139
  health 27–9

imbalance 9, 27, 29, 89
increasing 11, 29, 50
Kyo and Jitsu 88–92
matter relationship 13
meaning 1, 2, 6, 7, 12
source 13–14
subtle bodies 14–17
Yin and Yang 94–6
etheric body 14–15, 16,
17, 109
exercise 113, 115, 116,
119, 121, 122, 139–46
eyes, problems 42, 134,
135, 136, 138

face 80–3, 133
fatigue 133, 134, 135, 136,
138, 139
fear 110, 136
feedback 54, 83, 86
feet
in diagnosis 109, 113,
120, 121–2
problems 135
technique 65, 66–8, 132
fever 133, 137
Fu 21, 22
full-body treatment
58–84, 127

Gall Bladder 22
in diagnosis 111, 112,
117, 119, 121, 123,
124
Meridian 24, 25, 26,
121, 146
Tsubos 130–2, 136–7
Governing Vessel 23, 25,
130–2, 137–8

haemorrhoids 133, 138
hands
in diagnosis 125
problems 133, 134
technique 40, 74–6
Tsubos 130
Hara 45, 46, 47, 49, 51,
71, 111, 122
hay fever 134
head 80–3, 114–15, 131
head centre 46

headaches 26
after Shiatsu 42, 43
treatment 133, 134,
135, 136, 137, 138
health
definition 27–9
serious problems 41
Yin and Yang 98–9
Heart 22
centre 45, 46
Chakra 19, 20, 45, 111,
112, 123, 124
in diagnosis 111, 112,
115, 121, 123, 124,
125
Meridian 23, 24, 26,
124, 144
problems 134, 136, 138
Tsubos 130–2, 134
Heart Governor
Meridian 24, 26, 145
Organ 21–2
Tsubos 130–2, 136
hemiplegia 133
hips 68–9, 113, 114, 137
hives 134
hormonal system 23, 98
hypertension 133, 136
hysteria 134

impotence 135, 136, 137
infertility 135, 137
insomnia 134, 135, 136
Intestines
see also Large and
Small Intestines
in diagnosis 113, 119,
120, 121, 122
problems 133, 134
irritability 134
itching 134, 137

Jitsu 88–92, 120, 121, 124,
125, 128, 139, 140

Ki
see also Energy
definition 6, 7, 12
directing 32–5, 47, 50
imbalance 116, 117
perceiving 12, 14, 30–2

strengthening 138
Kidneys 2, 21, 22
in diagnosis 110, 111,
112, 113, 117, 119,
120, 121, 125
Meridian 24, 26, 120,
144
problems 135, 136, 137,
138
Tsubos 130–2, 136
knees 69, 114, 119–20,
137, 138
Kyo 88–92, 115, 117, 120,
121, 124, 128, 139, 140

lactation problems 137
Large Intestine 22
in diagnosis 111, 112,
115, 117
Meridian 25, 26, 141–2
Tsubos 126, 130–2, 133
legs
in diagnosis 111, 113,
114, 119–20
problems 134, 135, 137
technique 64–9, 130
Life Energy see Energy
Liver 21, 22
in diagnosis 111, 112,
117, 119, 121, 123,
124
Meridian 23, 24, 26,
121, 146
Tsubos 130–2, 137
lumbago 137
Lungs 22
in diagnosis 111, 112,
115, 116–17, 121
Meridian 23, 24, 26,
141–2
problems 134, 135, 138
Tsubos 130–2, 133

Makko-ho exercises
139–46
mastitis 137
menstrual problems 118,
134, 135, 136
mental body 15–16, 109
Meridians 23–6
definition 6, 8, 23

etheric body 15, 17
exercises 139–46
Kyo and Jitsu 88
Tsubos 126
migraine 43, 136
mucus, after Shiatsu 42
muscle tension 26, 41, 137

nausea 136
neck
  in diagnosis 114–15
  problems 133, 135, 136,
    137
  technique 77–9
neuralgia 133, 134
nose 133, 135, 137

Organs 15, 19, 21–3, 98
Orgone Energy *see*
  Energy
Oriental diagnosis 108–25
Oriental medicine 2, 6–8,
  9, 13, 17, 93

pain 42, 92, 116, 117–18,
  135, 136
pancreas 21, 110, 111,
  112, 119, 123, 124
personal power 111, 117,
  123
pharyngitis 133
pneumonia 135
Prana *see* Energy
pregnancy 40, 41, 128,
  133, 135, 137
pressure 6, 58, 59, 90–1,
  128
prolapsed anus or vagina
  138

relaxation 41, 83, 146
reproductive system
  in diagnosis 111, 112,
    118, 119, 120, 125
  problems 134, 135, 138
rheumatism 137

Sacral Chakra 19, 20, 111,
  112, 119
sciatica 135, 137
seiza 47, 48
sexual energy 111, 112,
  118, 119, 135
Shiatsu
  basic principles 50–7
  benefits 10–11
  effects 41–4
  history 6–7
  preliminary exercises
    45–57
  preparations for 38–40,
    58
  role today 8–11
  techniques 58–84
  varying treatment
    86–91
  when not to give 40–1,
    128, 133, 135, 137
shoulders
  in diagnosis 114,
    115–16, 117
  problems 133, 134, 136,
    137
  technique 40, 61–2
  Tsubos 126
shyness 136
sinusitis 133, 136, 138
Small Intestine 22
  in diagnosis 111, 112,
    117, 122
  Meridian 25, 26, 144
  problems 135
  Tsubos 130–2, 134
Solar Plexus Chakra 19,
  20, 111–12, 117, 123
speech problems 137
spiritual channel 17–21
Spleen 21, 22
  in diagnosis 110, 111,
    112, 113, 117, 119,
    123, 124
  Meridian 24, 26, 142–3
  Tsubos 130–2, 134
Stomach 21, 22, 138
  in diagnosis 110, 111,
    112, 113, 117, 119,
    123, 124

Meridian 24, 25, 26,
  142–3
  Tsubos 130–2, 133–4
stretches 52, 58, 91,
  139–46
subtle body system 14–17
Subtle Energy *see* Energy
Sushumna 17–21

teachers 1, 3, 147, 151
tension 110, 113–14, 117
thinking 26, 114, 137
throat 133, 134, 138
Throat Chakra 19, 20, 45,
  111, 112, 124
tiredness 42, 139
tonsilitis 133
toothache 126, 133, 134,
  136
touch 6, 10, 127
training schools 11, 147,
  151
Triple Heater
  Meridian 25, 26, 145
  Organ 21–2
  Tsubos 130–2, 136
Tsubos 8, 23, 27, 88,
  126–38

unconscious 110, 133

varicose veins 40
Vital Energy *see* Energy
vomiting 136

weight 50–7, 58, 59
Western medicine 7, 8–9,
  13, 17
wrists 125, 133

*Yellow Emperor's Classic
  of Internal Medicine* 6
Yin and Yang 94–102

Zang 21, 22